How Do You Doo?
Everybody Pees & Poops!

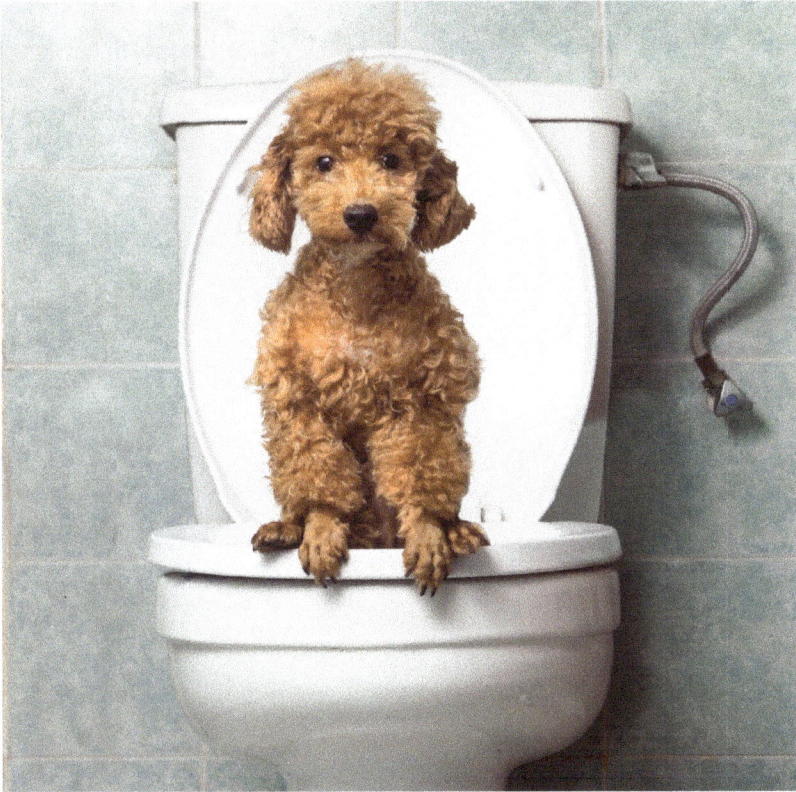

Nancy Cetel, MD
Joseph Weiss, MD

ISBN-13: 978-1-943760-06-0

Cover photo: copyright Shutterstock/ThamKC

DEDICATION

This book is dedicated to all of the parents, caregivers, and children who, for better or for worse, survive the toilet training process with their sense of humor and wonder intact.

CONTENTS

Chapter One

Training Parents for Potty Time

Toilet or potty training is the process of training a young child to use the toilet for peeing (urination) and pooping (defecation). The process requires cooperation and understanding between child and caregiver, and the best techniques use positive reinforcement, not punishment.

Cultural and societal factors play a surprisingly large role in determining the age when bowel and bladder control should be achieved. Being toilet trained at twelve months is expected for some tribes in Africa, while in the United States twenty-four to thirty-six months is more of the norm, with some efforts beginning at about eighteen months. Most children control their bowel before their bladder, and girls are usually more advanced than boys. Bed wetting at night (enuresis) may be the last challenge of toilet training to master, and nighttime dryness is usually achieved by the age of five or six in the US.

This is a much later age than seen in many other cultures. A parent or caregiver can have an advantage in the toilet training process if they are aware of and recognize the nonverbal clues and signs that many children exhibit as they have an internal urge to pee or poop. The most common finding if they have a need to pee is that they squirm, move or dance around, rocking from one foot to the other. Facial expressions of distraction and frustration may also be recognized.

The prompt offering of the potty seat and toilet time allows the need for peeing to be successfully achieved, with the bonus of giving an opportunity for positive reinforcement. The signs of the need to poop can be similar to peeing, but with the facial appearance of imminent straining. Once the straining and holding of breath begins, the time get to, and on the potty, is usually too late. If you can get there to catch some of the poop, and even right after the poop, it is still a good opportunity to offer positive reinforcement that the child is getting closer to the goal of depositing the poop in its proper place.

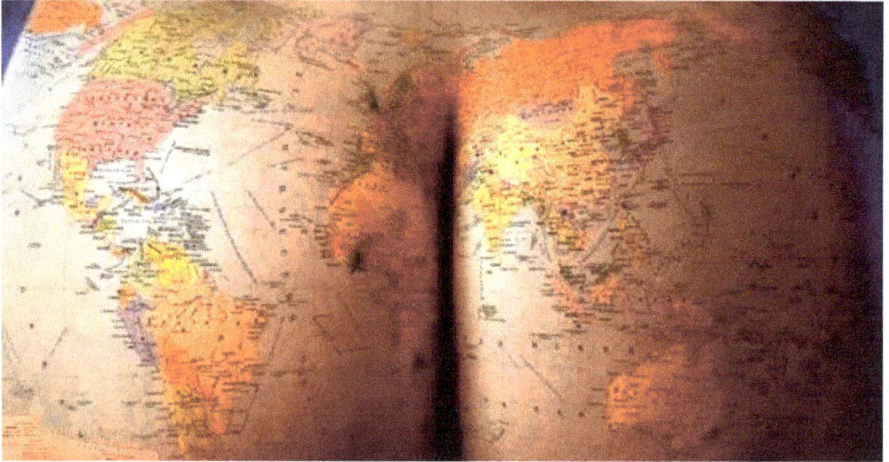

Toilet training practices and age of achievement vary around the world. The U.S. lags behind, and this generates enormous profits for the disposable diaper companies and extra burdens on waste management. Other countries start toilet training much earlier than in the US. In some cultures and societies infants and young children do not use diapers. Without the diapers to hide the evidence, the parent or caregiver is more observant of the child peeing and pooping. They quickly learn to recognize the child's nonverbal signs and communication of the need to pee and poop, and use that to initiate a visit to the potty or toilet. This natural and positive reinforcement leads to rapid toilet training.

In Vietnam potty training starts at birth, and infants are usually trained for urination by nine months of age! The technique is based on nonverbal communication, with the baby learning to associate its urination with a whistling sound the mother makes each time that it pees. With experience, the special whistling sound reminds the baby to urinate. They can generally take care of all their toileting needs by the age of two.

The age of toilet training has been delayed over the last several generations in the US. In the 1900's the majority of children in the US were toilet trained by age two, with training beginning before twelve months. It is not unusual for toilet training to now be delayed to an age of three years. The main instigator has been an unproven concern that toilet training initiated too early may lead to psychological issues with the start of toilet training now commonly delayed to eighteen months. With the enormous profits generated by increasing the time children spend in diapers, it would not be surprising if the disposable diaper companies funded or promoted distribution of the psychological studies supporting delayed toilet training. Perhaps new research showing the psychological issues related to delayed toilet training would allow the US to catch up with the potty progress of the rest of the world.

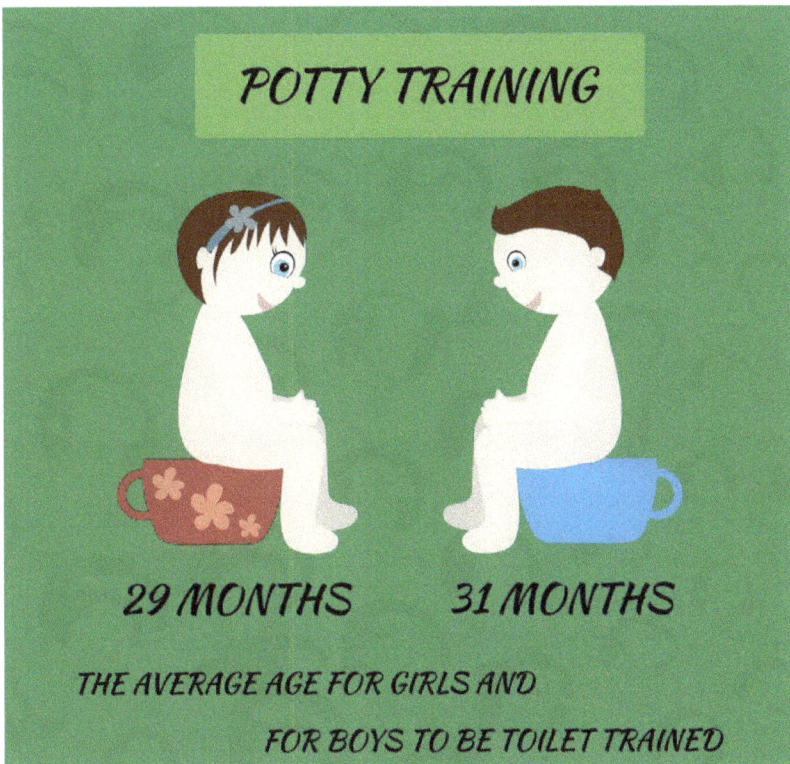

POTTY TRAINING

29 MONTHS   31 MONTHS

THE AVERAGE AGE FOR GIRLS AND
FOR BOYS TO BE TOILET TRAINED

Shutterstock Rusana Mishchenko

The ability to have two way communicate with the child is very important in the toilet training process. Although the ability to fully understand the child's verbal communication is optimal, nonverbal communication can also be very effective. It is recognized that preschool potty training envy will often encourage children to try to catch up with their preschool classmates who are potty trained and more independent. Parents may find this motivation useful in encouraging their children to progress if they are ready. Besides, if they can be toilet trained at an earlier age like elsewhere in the world, the thousands of dollars saved on disposable diapers could be contributed to a sizable college education trust fund for their future financial benefit. Of course there is also an environmental benefit by reducing the impact on landfills and pollution.

The potty selected should be at comfortable child height, and kept close to where the child spends most of its time. It should be readily portable, easy to clean, and attractive to the child so that he or she associates it with a positive activity. Perhaps the child has an interest in seeing it decorated with playful and fun stickers, or has their name on it. The ability to respond promptly by having the child sit on the potty at the early signs of needing to pee or poop is a priority.

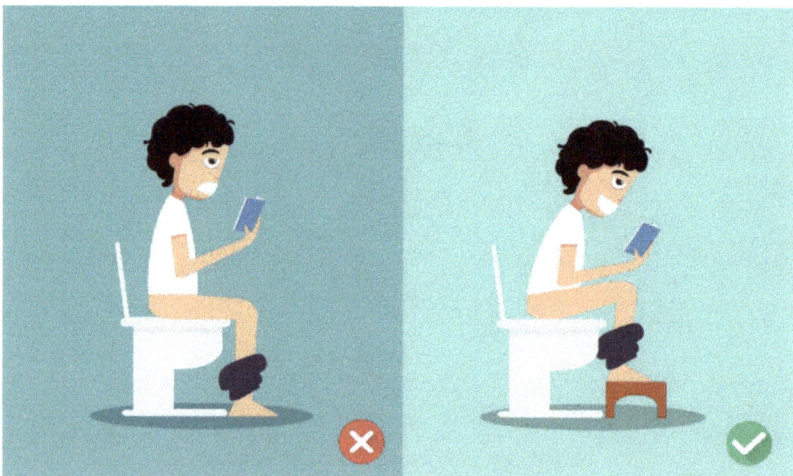

Shutterstock jehsomwang

Chapter Two

Pooping a Bowel Movement

Defecation is the act of a bowel movement, often referred to simply by its abbreviated initials BM. It is the elimination of digestive waste material expelled from the gastrointestinal tract via the rectum and anus. The digestive waste is called by many different names and terms. The proper medical term is feces, but it is commonly known as poop, crap, excrement, shit, droppings, turd, and dozens of euphemisms, alternate words used to avoid those considered offensive or embarrassing.

The stimulus to defecate, which results in the sense and urge to defecate, is the stretching and distention of the rectum or sigmoid colon by feces. The ability to recognize and interpret this sensation is one of the challenges faced by the child, whose life so far has been a series of learning experiences. They have already achieved so much, perhaps having mastered the use of their limbs and fingers, crawling, and even walking. Learning to recognize internal sensations and express them is within their abilities as they communicate hunger, thirst, sleepiness, humor, and love.

One physiologic reflex that the adult can use to help the child recognize the internal urge to go to the toilet is called the gastrocolic reflex. This fancy term describes the known phenomenon that eating food can trigger the need to empty the bowels. Many recognize that baby's will often have a bowel movement during or immediately after a feeding. The same reflex continues throughout childhood and in some continues on to adulthood. It is not uncommon for people to find that eating breakfast or having a morning beverage such as coffee will stimulate a bowel movement. It is possible to use this reflex signal to advantage by encouraging a child to sit on the potty for a brief time after the morning meal to encourage a bowel movement and try to establish a pattern and regularity.

For those parents who are anal-retentive and want to know more about the mechanism and physiology of defecation, this next paragraph is for you. For the rest who need no in depth explanation of how the miracle of pooping occurs, you can gleefully skip on to the next paragraph. Defecation is actually a complex reflex coordination of neuromuscular activity. It requires the relaxation of the puborectalis muscle to allow the straightening the anorectal angle, which is normally at a ninety-degree angle. This induces the involuntary relaxation of the internal anal sphincter. The relaxation of the internal anal sphincter creates a strong urge to defecate. The external anal sphincter, which is under voluntary control, then contracts to prevent defecation until it is voluntarily released to allow the defecation process to proceed.

Once the external anal sphincter is relaxed, colonic contractions along with increased intra-abdominal pressure by performance of the Valsalva maneuver (attempting to exhale against a closed epiglottis), propel the feces out of the rectum via the anus. Learning to control the external anal sphincter is thus a major key to the toilet training required for bowel control. Learning how to perform the Valsalva maneuver is a natural instinct, as is the contraction of the abdominal muscles to increase intraabdominal pressure to expel the feces.

Anorectal Angle

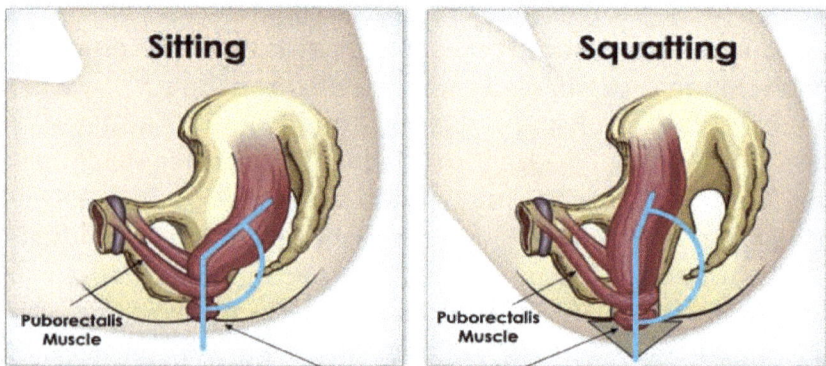

Squatting is the most natural defecation posture.

The frequency range of normal bowel movements is variable, and can range from two bowel movements per day to once per week. It is often dependent on diet, activity, and social habit. The squatting position is the most natural position to assume allows greater ease with defecation and toilet training. Using Western style sitting toilets, as opposed to squat toilets found in non-Western locales, is much more challenging. It can be very difficult to defecate if the feet cannot comfortably reach the ground, as commonly occurs in young children sitting on an adult toilet. An elevated footrest to allow the firm placement of the feet, so that the legs and thighs are flexed and bent at the knees, can greatly assist in the ease of elimination for both children and adults.

The ability to flex at the knees allows a position similar to squatting on a sitting toilet, which relaxes the muscles to allow straightening of the anorectal angle. The straightening of this angle is very important, and required for normal defecation to take place. If your child is also spending part if their day in a preschool, child care facility, or in the home of another, take the time to go with your child to the other toilet facility to make sure it is comfortable, especially the ability to place the child's feet on a secure setting such as floor or footstool.

The use of a small potty has the advantage of the child being able to keep their feet on the ground for better balance and a more squat-like posture. Some water can be placed in the potty bowl to ease cleaning and reduce the smell of feces. The child can watch or assist in emptying their potty into the adult toilet for flushing. A natural transition to an adult toilet can be undertaken when they are ready. Regular adult toilets have an opening that is normally too large and frightening for a child, yet may be used if a secure child seat adapter is provided.

Their fear of the toilet is not unjustified; as American adults suffer forty thousand toilet related injuries per year. Keep in mind that transition to an adult toilet, even with a child seat adapter, requires another important consideration. Difficulty with the seated position on an adult toilet is common as their feet often cannot reach the floor. Since they can no longer brace their feet, the squat like position to straighten the anorectal angle is lost and defecation becomes very difficult. If the cause is not recognized and corrected the adult may become frustrated that it is taking the child so long to defecate.

The adult may not realize that without the child being able to brace their feet and apply resistance that they are also unable to generate the intra-abdominal pressure needed to promote defecation. A footstool built into the child seat, or a separate footstool at the appropriate height, can be a great help the initiation of a bowel movement and can accelerate toilet training.

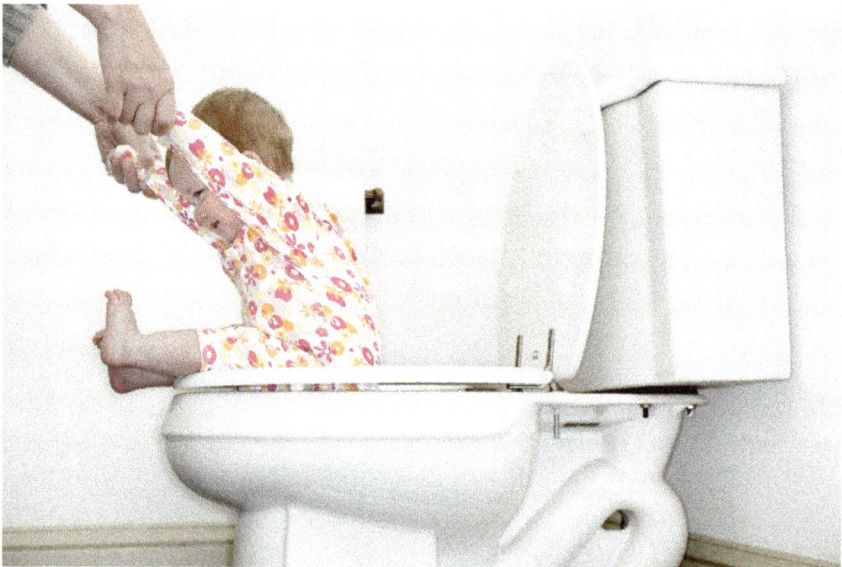

Some children are frightened by the rush of water and noise generated by the flush, especially if not a low flow or quiet toilet. In that case it may be best to wait to flush until the child is out of the bathroom. Other children seem to enjoy the activity of flushing, and see it as a reward for their success in using the potty. Allowing the child to recognize their accomplishments self-reinforces good behavior. The poop itself is often referred to in cute terms, such as little fishes about to swim from the toilet bowl pool with their friends, to the river, lake, ocean, or other large body of water.

The successful pee or poop in the potty or toilet can be rewarded with verbal and mincer all expressions of approval. The use of stickers, gold stars, and nominal symbols of success are also reasonable. The reward of food or candy should be discouraged, as society has more than enough of an obesity issue with food considered as a reward and means of gratification.

Accidents will happen, and It is important to avoid punishment or harsh verbal or nonverbal displays of disappointment when they inevitably occur. Toilet training is a learning process, and the child learns best in a supportive and encouraging environment. Accidents and setbacks should be expected, and used as a learning experience to encourage efforts of the child to improve and reduce future episodes as much as possible.

The limiting of drinking fluids a few hours before bedtime, and encouraging peeing just before going to bed, will help the child stay dry through the night. There are many books for children that help to inform and entertain them (as well as the reader) about the natural elimination functions and process. Although poop is more challenging than peeing, keep a positive attitude about is importance and that it is part of nature.

While the aroma and hygiene aspects of poop leave a lot to be desired, it is best to just be matter of fact with a touch of light humor. Let the child know that it is normal waste, and it is good that it goes where it belongs in the toilet and not in diapers or underwear. After bathroom hygiene is important and should be emphasized at the same time as toilet training. Wiping with wet wipes and then toilet paper from front to back is an important step to minimize the risk of urinary tract infections, especially in girls.

With boys there is the option of peeing while standing, and that is fine as long as they have mastered peeing sitting down and their balance is good. The young boy may observe its father, adult male, or older brother pee standing up and want to imitate this behavior. Standing on a footstool to pee into an adult toilet is not a great idea (especially for girls!), even with the adult there to make sure balance and aim are on target. Children with this experience may try this circus act on their own, and balance and hand-eye coordination have yet to be fully developed. Falling off the footstool facing a large open toilet bowl is more dangerous than the result of poor aim.

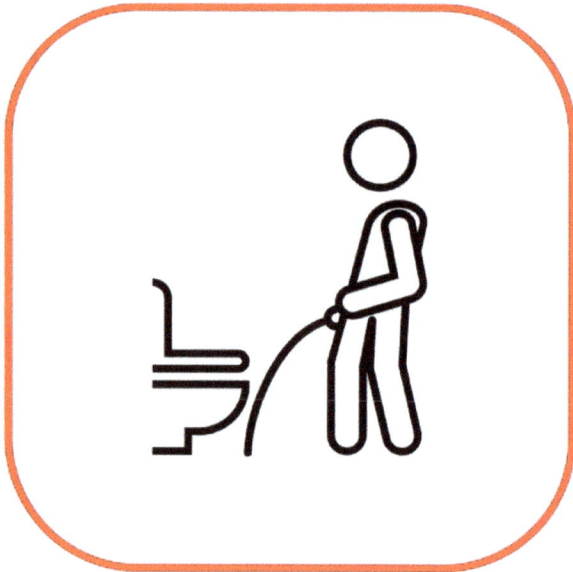

If you are a boy, one day you can stand and pee. Be sure you have good aim, like a dog aiming for a tree. Shutterstock/redline vector

The young boy standing technique is better mastered by peeing into a wide mouthed pail, and with time and experience, the potty is ready for target practice. Literal target practice is fine, and the child and caregiver often enjoys making the process a fun sporting event. Flushable disposable targets are especially made for this purpose, but cereals such as Cheerios,

Fruit Loops, etc. are handy inexpensive substitutes.

Speaking of animals, children are often delighted to discover that other animals and they are often very much alike. Seeing baby animals and their parents as a family, and sharing a need to eat, breath, drink, bathe, and yes, pee and poop can be reaffirming and encourage their interest in toilet habits. Sharing with the child that dog poop on the lawn is not a good behavior, may provide an opportunity to describe our social and cultural beliefs and behaviors. The following selection of photographs of various animals in the natural act can allow this book to serve as reading or potty entertainment and education, on animals, bodily processes, and the great adventure of life and learning.

For the reader that has an interest in learning much more about digestion and health, from major scientific advances such as the gut microbiome, genomics, and stem cells to nanotechnology and beyond, I have written a number of in depth books that are very informative and entertaining. For those who want their education and entertainment focused on the aspects of digestion rarely discussed, I have additional volumes on intestinal gas, scatology, and serious poop that are also full of fascinating information in an entertaining and colorfully well illustrated format.

Chapter Three

Animals Doo it Too!

ANIMALS HAVE TO POO TOO,
JUST LIKE YOU, THEY REALLY DOO!

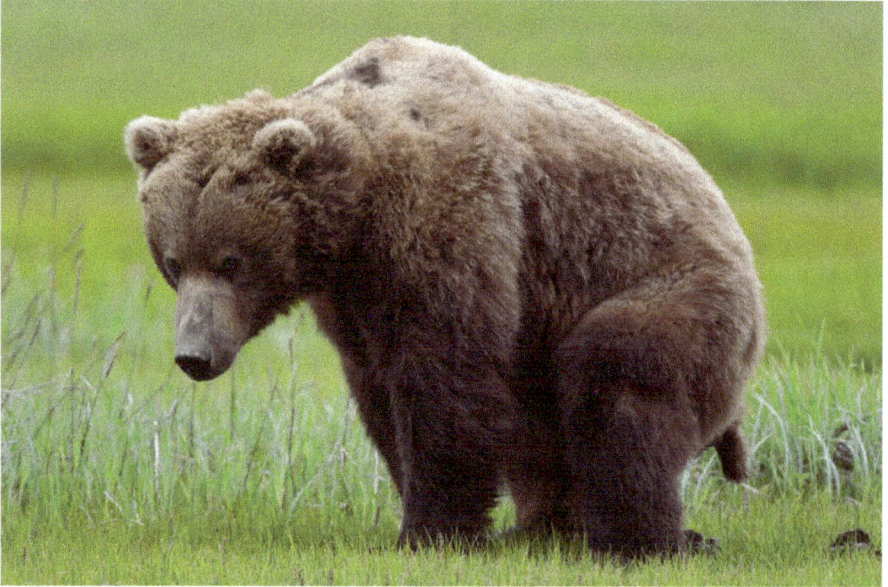

I have to bear down to poop!

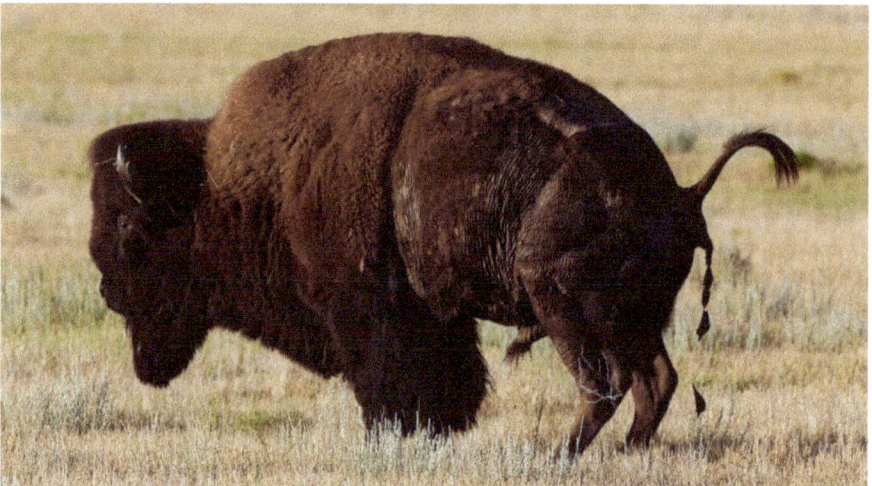

Be careful where you step, if walk in the fields where the buffalo roam!

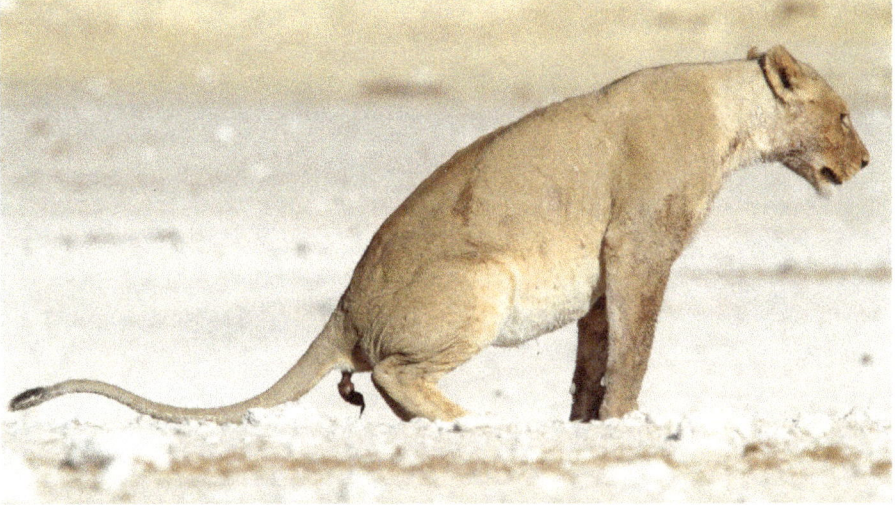

If I told you I didn't poop I be lyin', and lions don't do that!

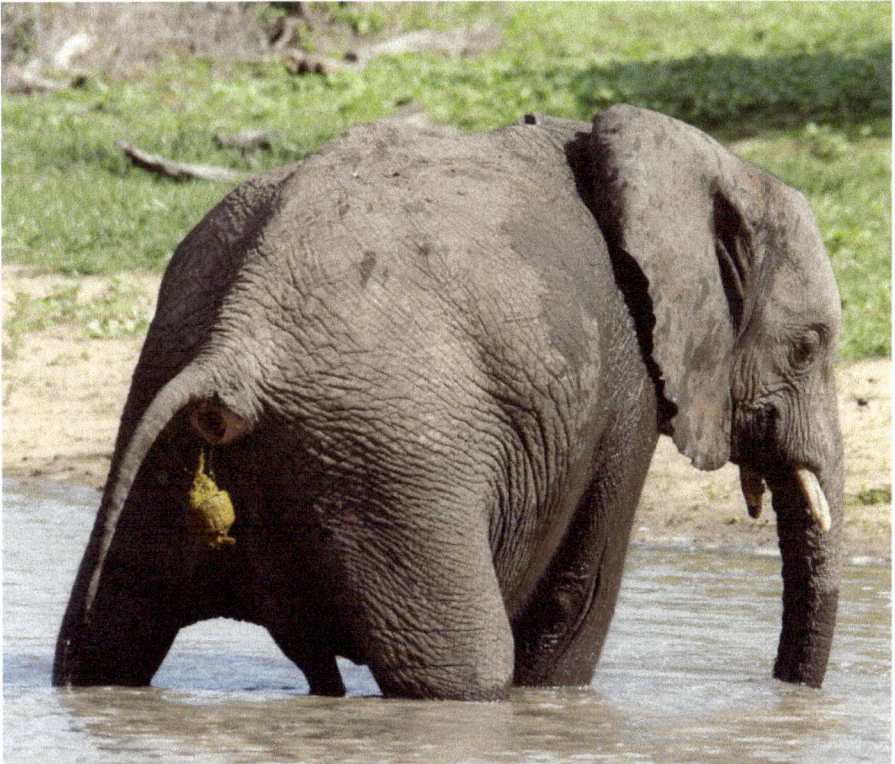

With my memory, I don't have to remember to flush in the river

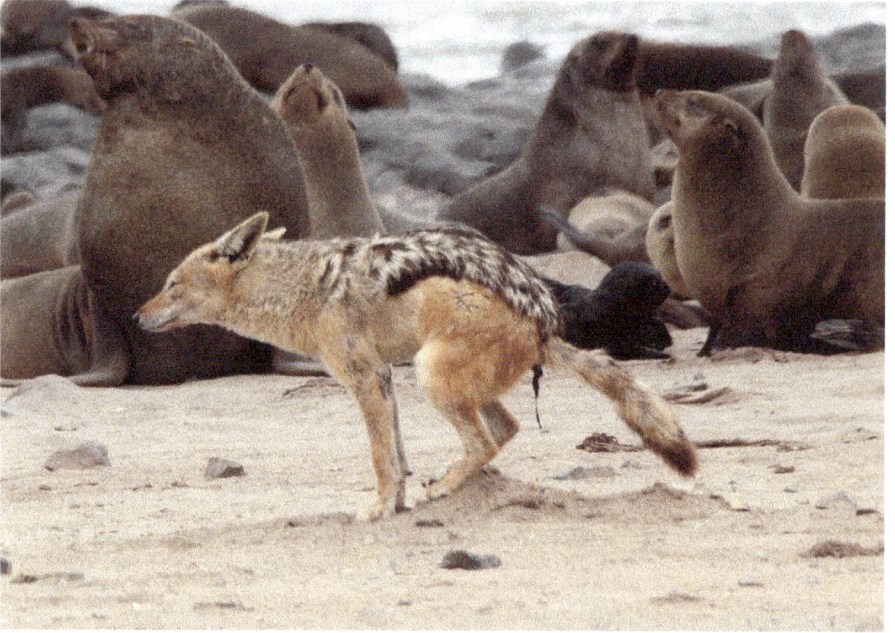

I was once in a litter, so I litter the beach with my scat!

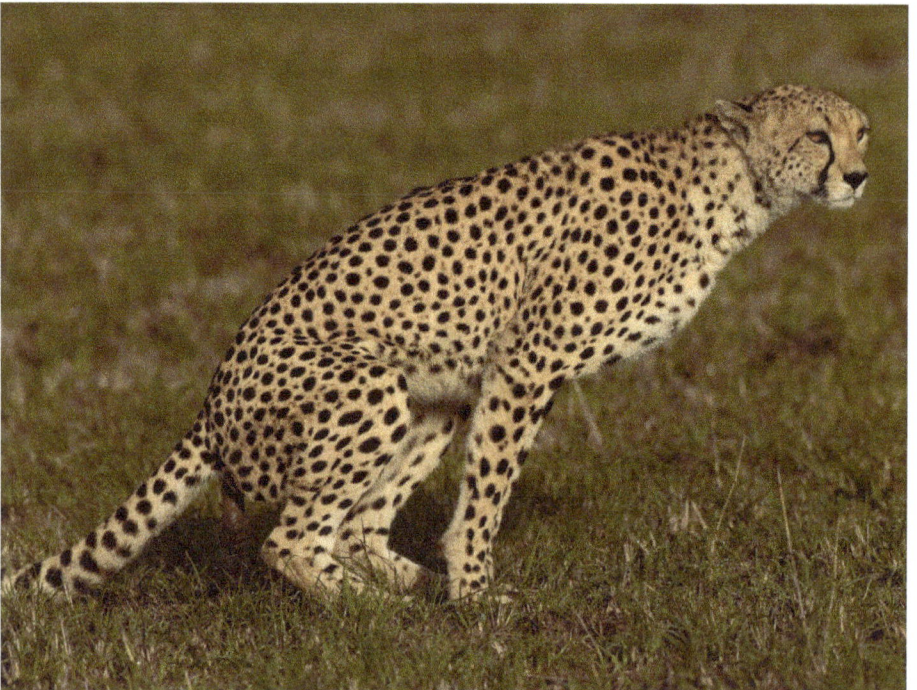

Do you spot a cheetah? You doo! This is a good spot to poop.

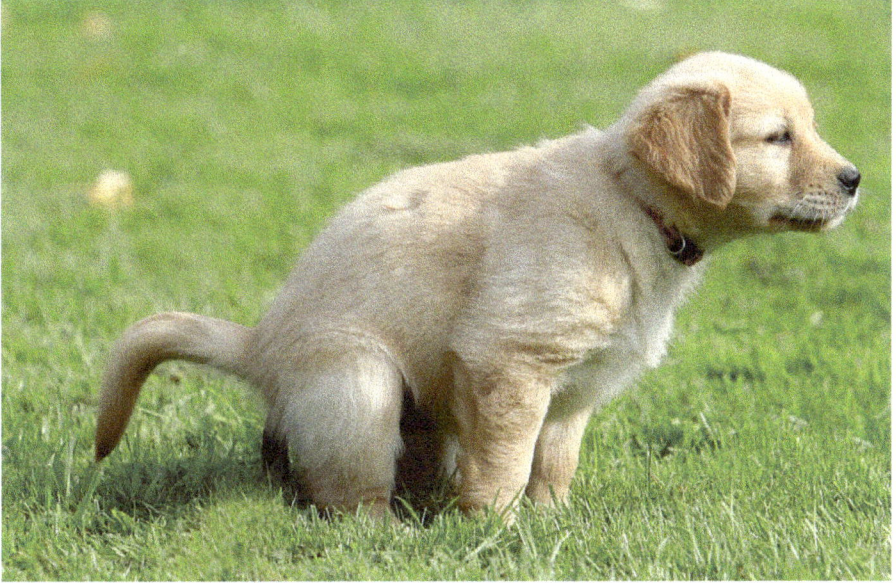

As a puppy I am cute no matter what I doo!

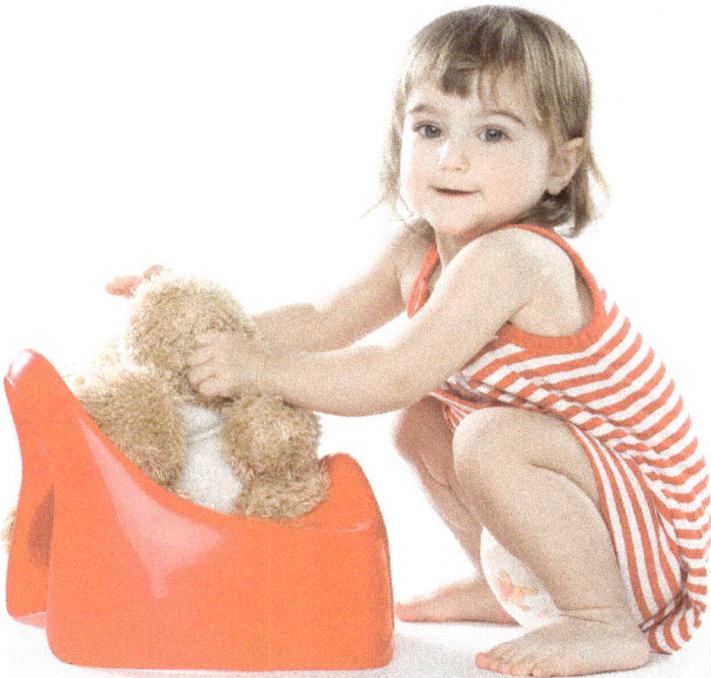

With potty training, diapers cost squat in our family budget!

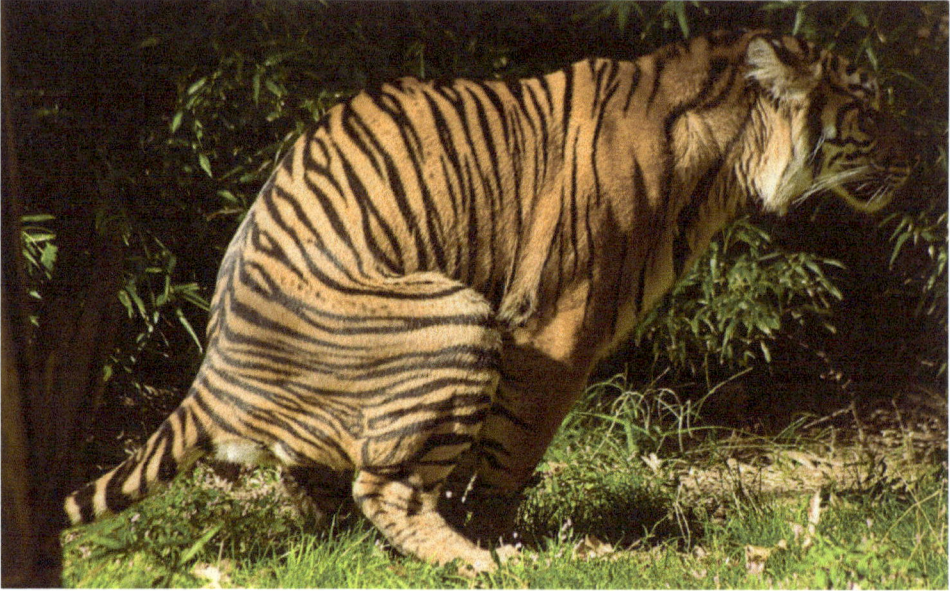

Animals of all stripes poop. Tiger Poop Juehua Yin Creative Commons License

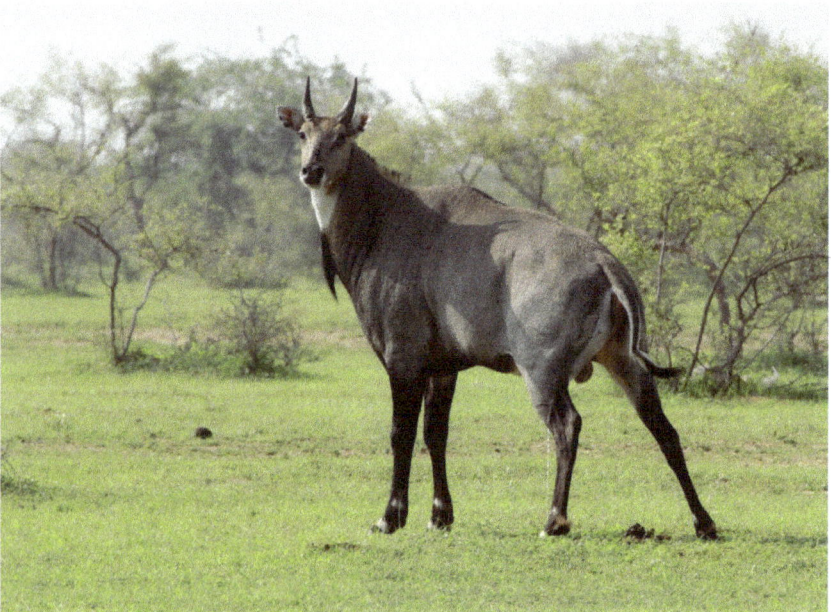

Antelopes Poop, and so do all of your other Aunties too. Shutterstock/Cat Downie

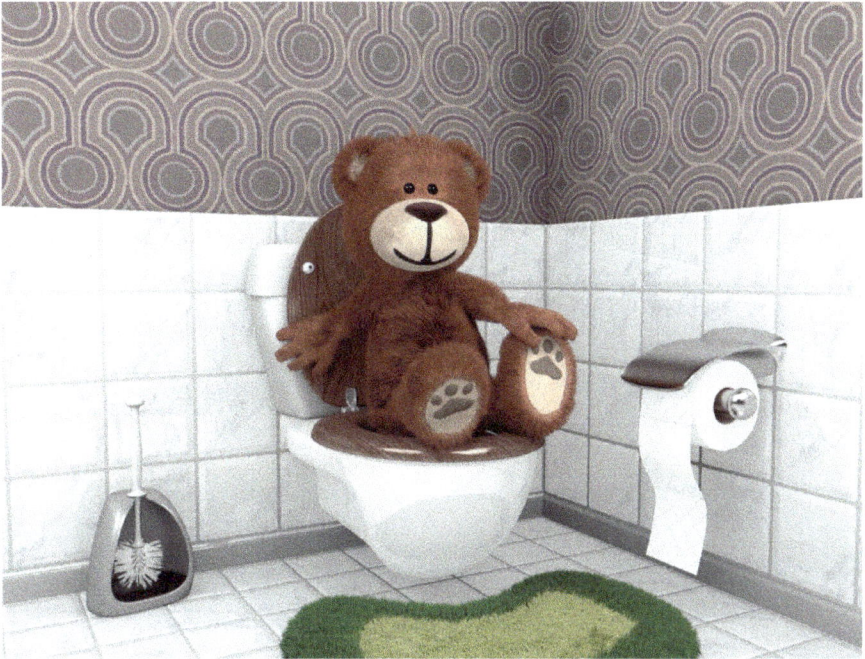

Teddy Bears and other pretend creatures like Winnie the Poo, might pretend to poop. Shutterstock/sarbiewski

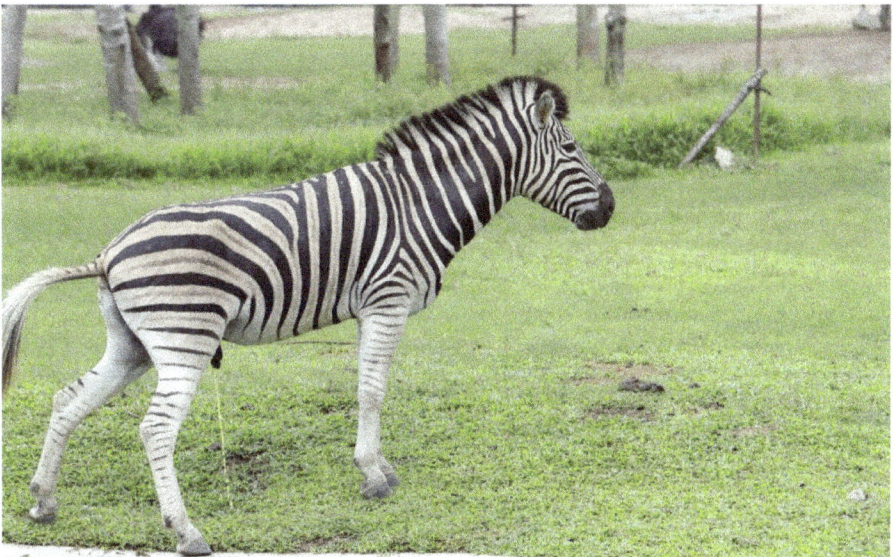

A zebra is another example that animals of all stripes peep and poop. Shutterstock/konmesa

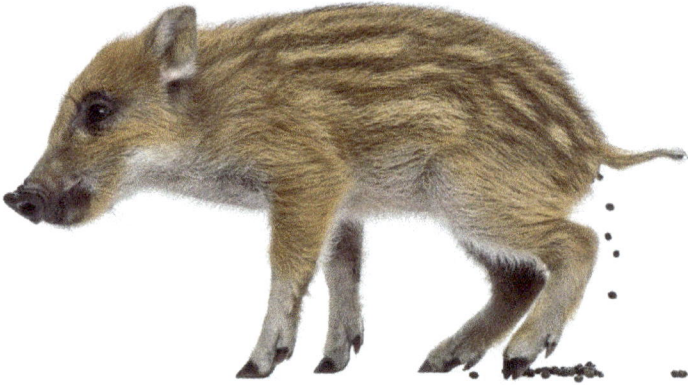

Even though a Boar can get bored, it is always exciting when it is time to poop. Wild Boar Piglet Poop/Eric Isselee

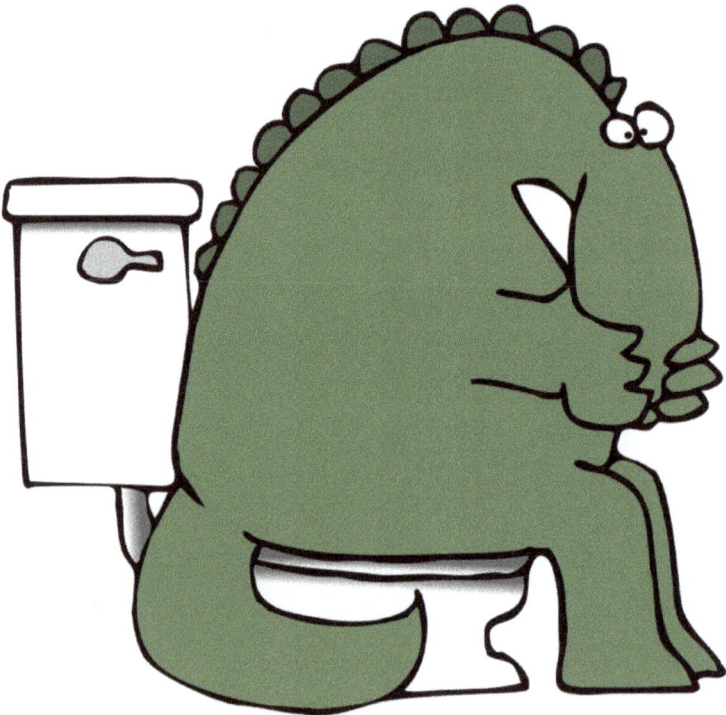

I was the largest animal on the planet when I roamed the Earth, but I am now extinct. My petrified poop is collected by archaeologists, and thank goodness it no longer stinks. Dinosaur Poop/Dennis Cox

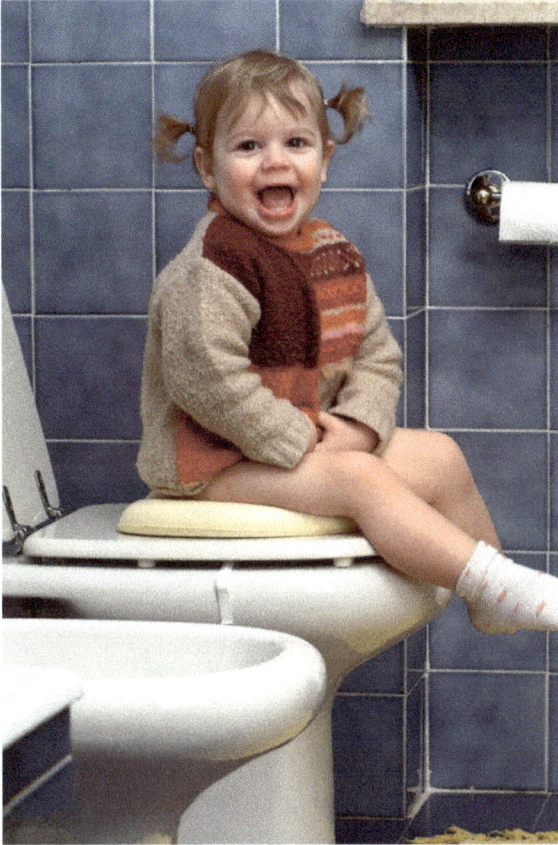

I am as proud as can be, I sit on the toilet when I have to poop or pee.
Shutterstock Maurizio Milanesio

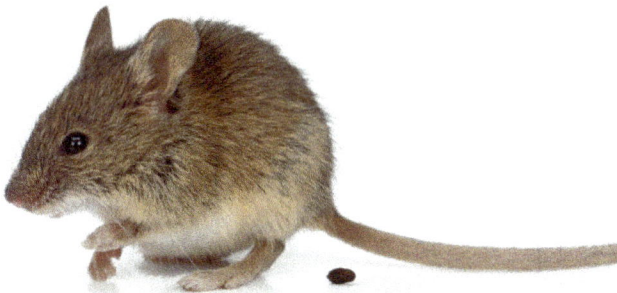

A mouse is so small, that the size of its poop is hardly anything at all. Mouse
Poop/Szasz-Fabian Jozsef

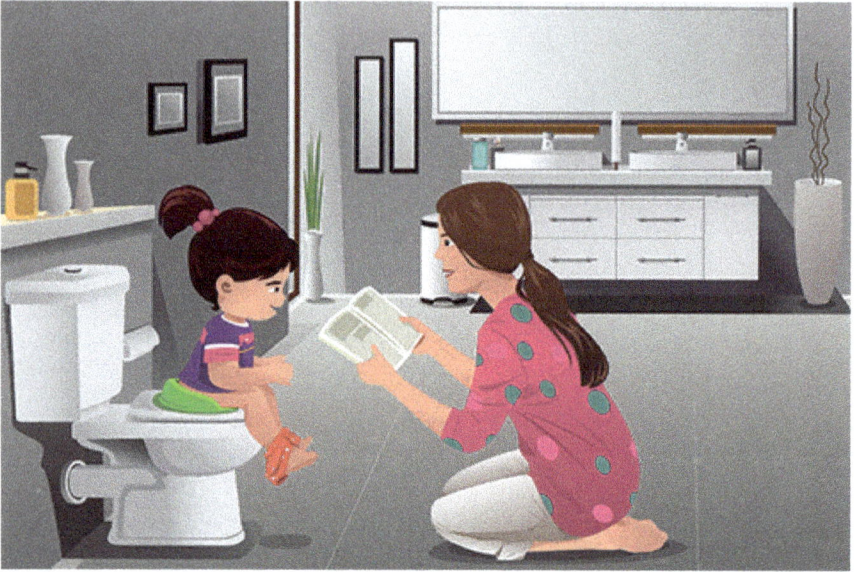

While I poop and pee, my mom reads to me. Shutterstock Artisticco

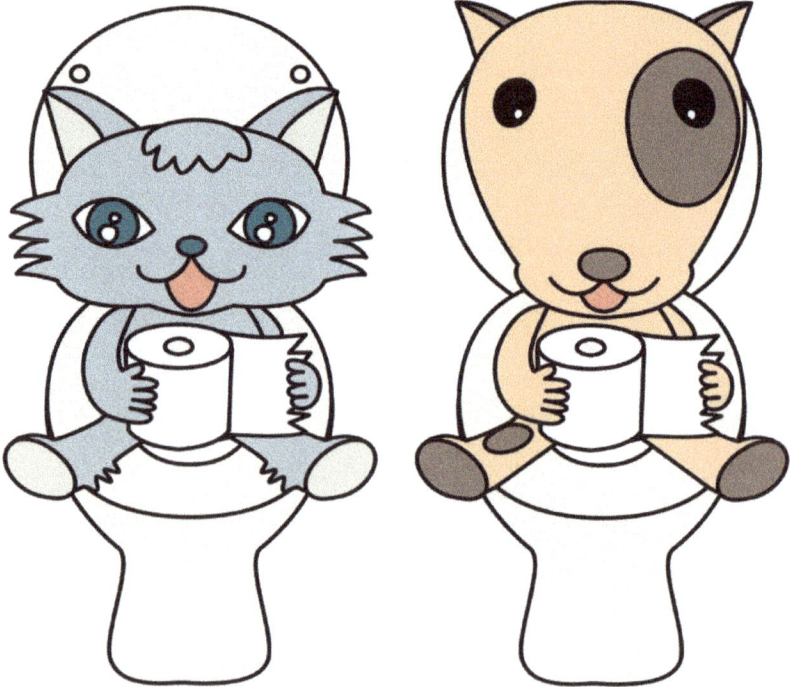

If you have a pet a dog or a cat, you know that no one wants to find scat. Cat & Dog Toilet/Moriko

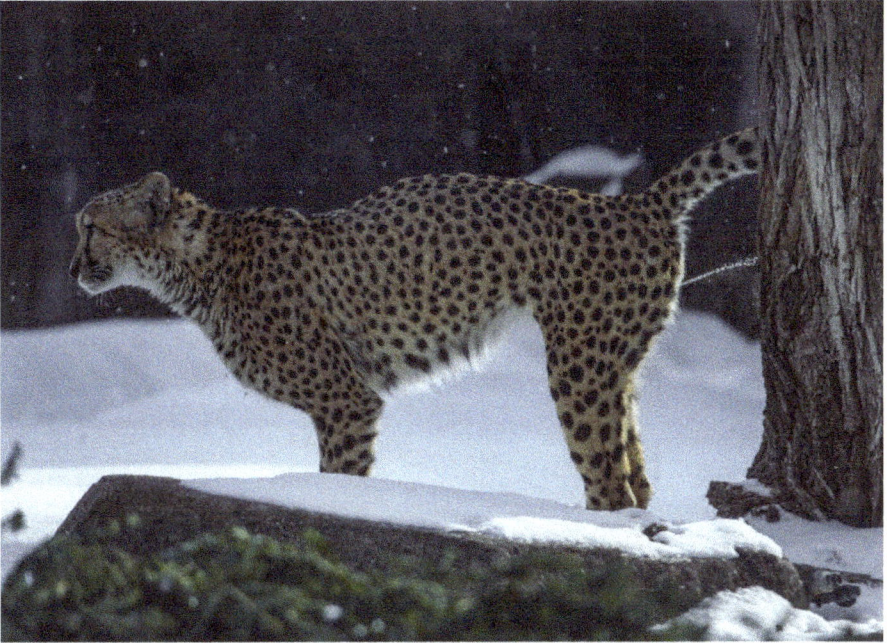

A cheetah would not cheat, it aims its pee at a tree. Cheetah Pee/Kris Wiktor

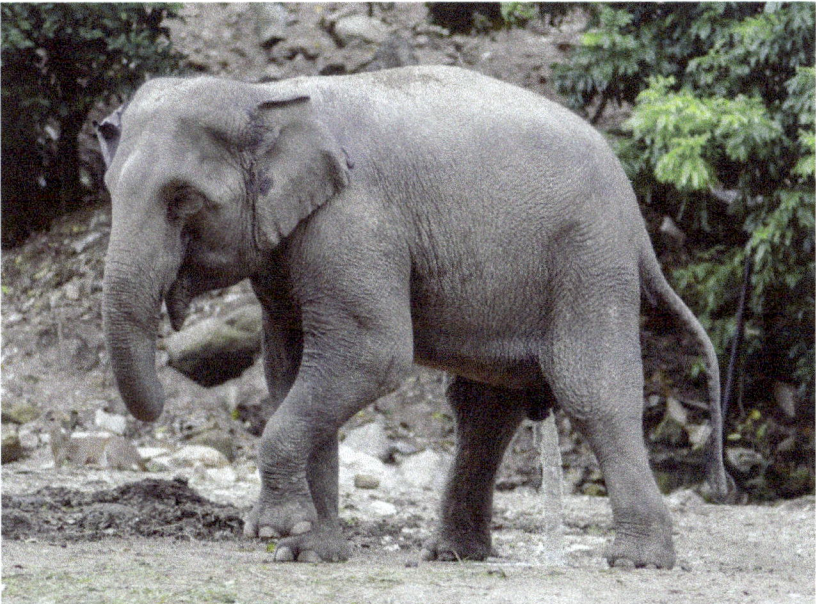

An elephant is a very big animal, and when it pees it leaves a big puddle. Elephant Pee/Piyathep

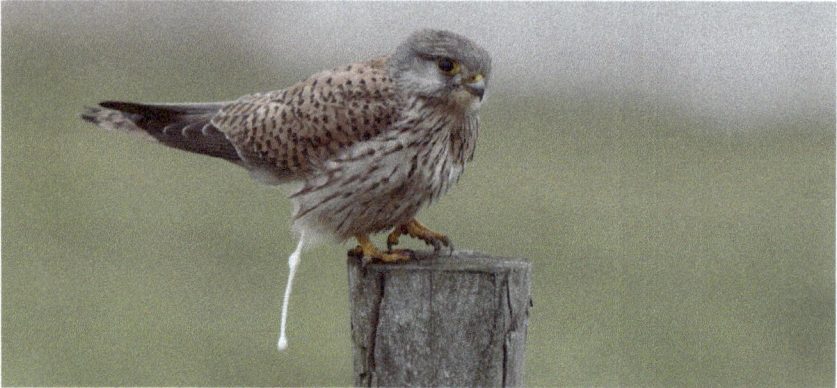

Guess what they sometimes call the poop of a bird? If you guessed right, you guessed turd. European Common Kestrel Bird Poop/Menno Schaefer

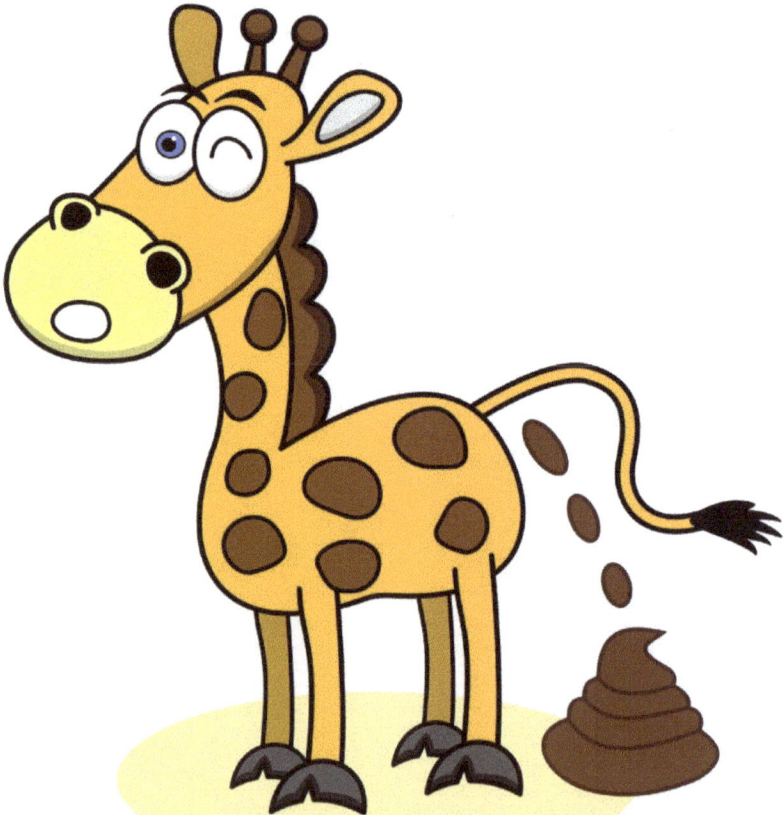

A giraffe is so tall that sometimes it has to stoop, of course it sometimes also has to poop. Giraffe Poop/Barkas

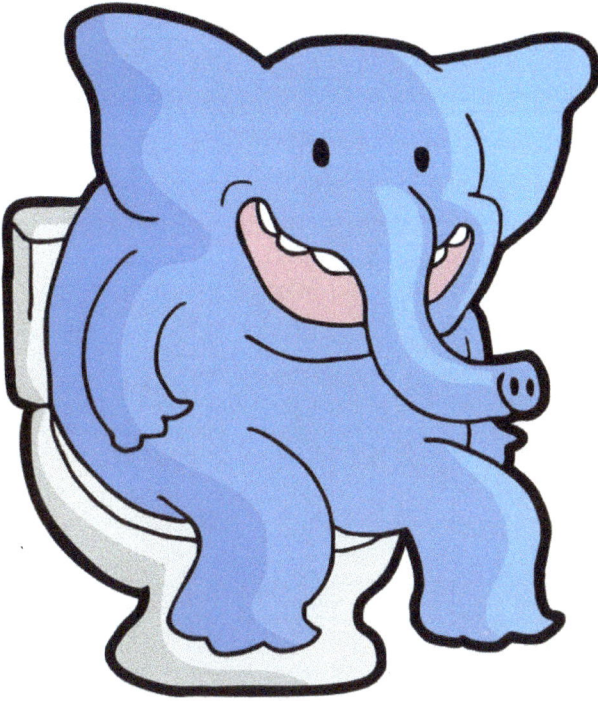

Sitting on a toilet is good way to poop and pee, but the toilet would probably tell someone as heavy as the elephant please don't sit on me.
Elephant Poop/Ratoca

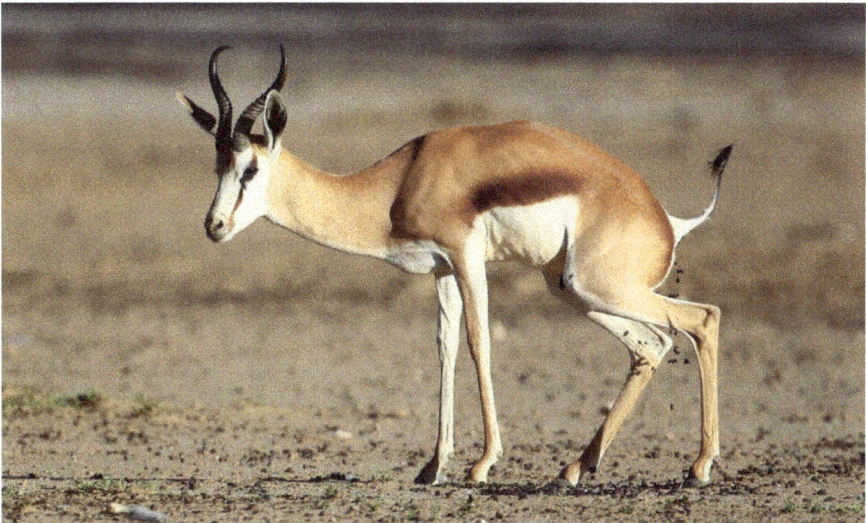

Every animal poops and pees, just like you and me, Springbuck Poop/JMx Images

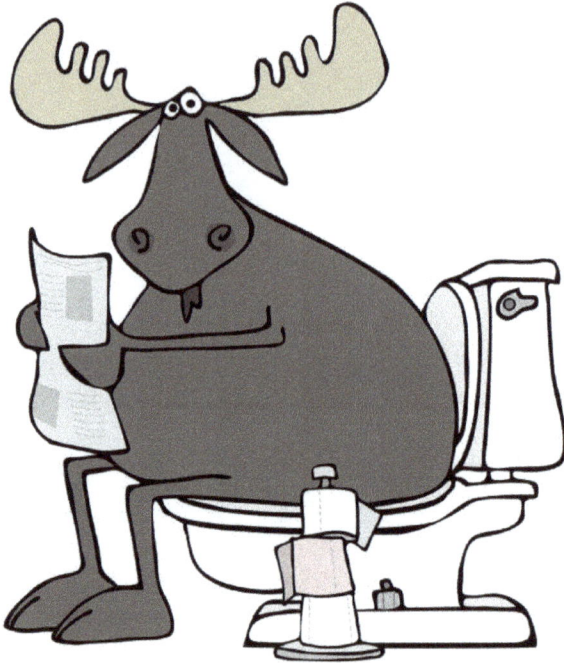

A moose is a big animal too, but it has to poop just like you. Moose Poop/Dennis Cox

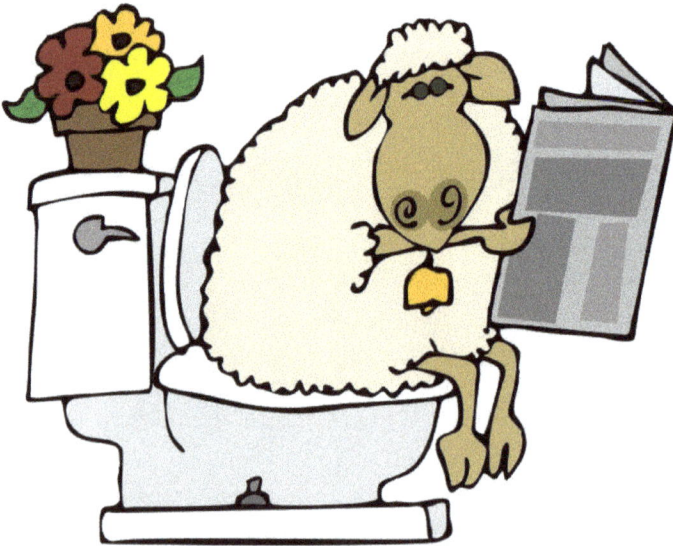

If you live on a sheep farm you know that we poop too, just like you. Sheep Poop/Dennis Cox

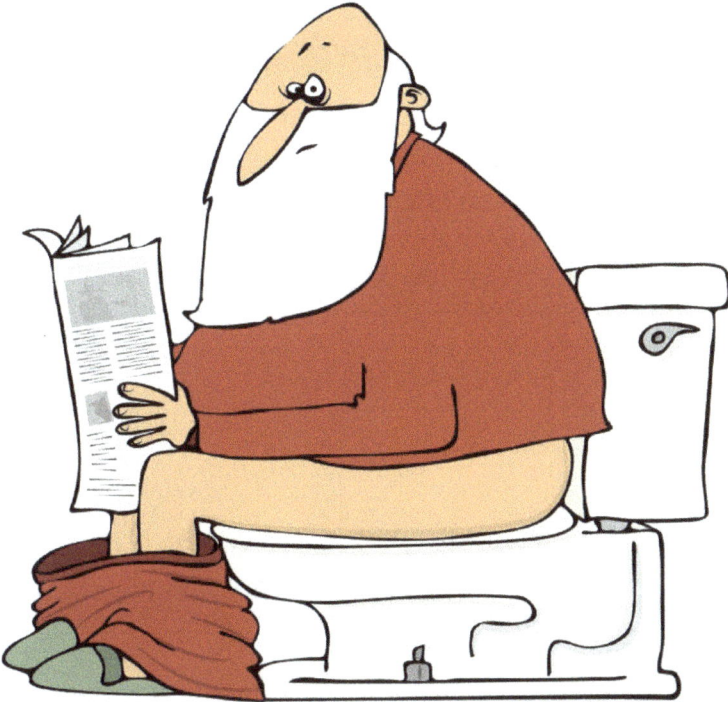

Just like the reindeer and Mrs. Claus, another person that has to poop is Santa Claus. Shutterstock/Dennis Cox

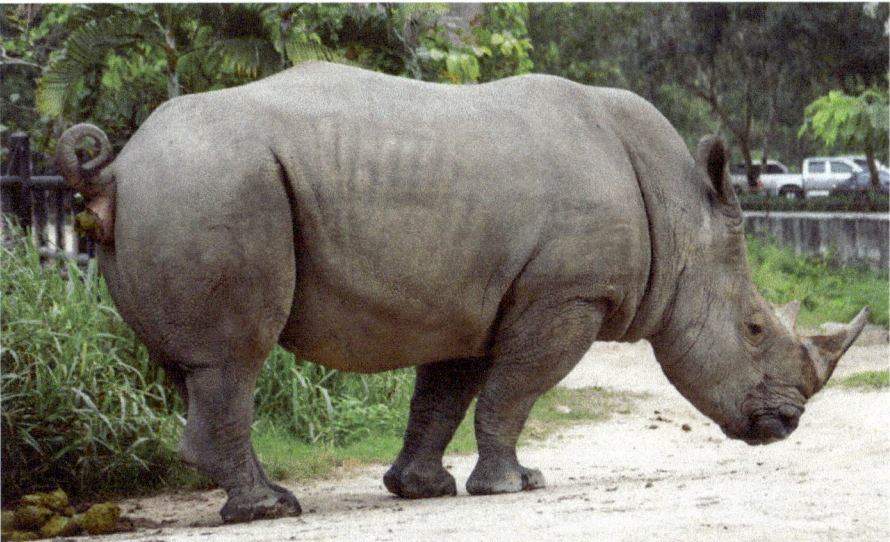

With poop this big, I know, it must be from a Rhino! Poop/krichie

Chapter Four

It Takes Guts, A Digest on Digestion

Perhaps the best analogy is to think of the digestive tract as the reverse of an assembly line, it serves as a disassembly line. A factory has a goal to be efficient and profitable, and may not win too many awards for architecture and beauty. So too with the digestive tract, the process has been refined over eons of evolution, yet still has its primitive origin and end products.

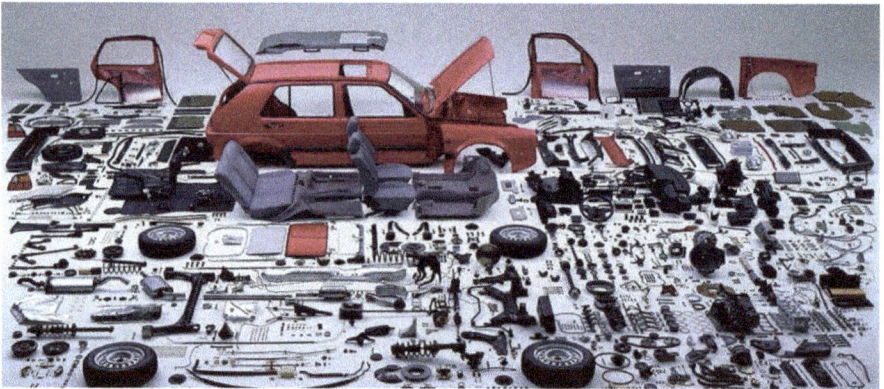

We begin the factory tour with a view much like you would get sitting in your car going through a car wash. Before you even go to the car wash, your brain has to make the conscious decision that that is what it wants to do. In the same manner, the brain begins the digestive process with the decision to satisfy its hunger call, or because an appetizing opportunity presents itself. When thinking about food and eating, the brain may release hormones and neurotransmitters, activate the secretion of saliva, and prime the release of gastric acid and digestive enzymes to prime and initiate the process of digestion.

Much like the water hoses and spray that greet your vehicle as you enter the beginning of the car wash tunnel, the entrance of food to the mouth receives a similar welcome. Jets of saliva are secreted from the ducts of the salivary glands located strategically around the oral cavity of the mouth. Saliva that is in the resting mouth is viscous and coats and protects the teeth and the inner surface of the mouth. The secreted saliva associated with eating or drinking is of a thinner waterier consistency. It has digestive enzymes including amylase to digest carbohydrates and lipase to digest fats.

1.Mouth

When food is chewed, saliva starts digesting carbohydrates.

2.Esophagus

Muscles, in a process called peristalsis, push the food down into your stomach.

3.Stomach

Everything is blended with digestive juices. Hydrochloric Acid kills bacteria. Enzymes break down proteins.

4. Liver

A green liquid called bile, which is stored in your liver, is secreted to break down fats.

5.Pancreas

Many kinds of digestive enzymes are made here.

6.Small Intestine

Food is mixed with bile from your liver and juices from your pancreas to be sent back to your liver for more processing.

7.Large Intestine

Indigestible food and water are processed, stored and dispersed.

8.Anus

Solid waste passes from the rectum in order to leave your body.

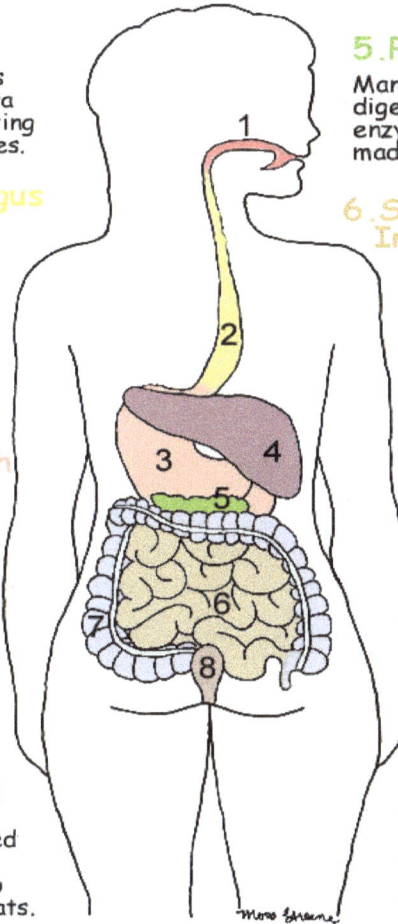

anatomy456.wordpress.com

If your carwash is as sophisticated as your digestive tract, it will have a crew to make sure your side mirrors are tucked in, and a prewash scrub of your tires and residue that would

otherwise be difficult for the machinery to access. The teeth, jaws, and tongue work together in a remarkable and powerful dance with very few of the missteps which would be the dance equivalent of stepping on toes, the biting of the tongue.
The food has to be processed into smaller more manageable portions than what is found on your plate. Your dining utensils are just the preliminary, as the teeth do the real work in preparing food for the process of digestion. The teeth are subdivided into specific categories that have unique functions. The incisors cut the food as you bite into an apple, the canines tear the food apart as you dig into your pastrami sandwich, and your molars crush and grind the salad and crunchy vegetables you have as a side dish. The grinding and crushing break the plant cell walls apart that would otherwise protect its internal nutritious content. They also increase the surface area for food to be exposed to digestive acid and enzymes.

The chewing process assures that the saliva and its active enzymes are well mixed with the increased surface area of the food. They begin the process of breaking down the carbohydrates and lipids into their essential components to ready them for further digestion and absorption. The saliva also moistens the food and lubricates it for the coordinated motion of the tongue, teeth, palate and pharynx. These muscles and organs work together to roll it into an easy to swallow food bolus. The muscles of the swallowing process include those that protect the larynx and airway. By having the epiglottis close off the passageway to the trachea, bronchi, and lungs, it prevents aspiration into the airways as the food and saliva swallows take place.

The coordinated action is developed with age, which is why small children should avoid foods, such as nuts, grapes, and larger oval or rounded candies. These foods, if misdirected into the airway, can lead to fatal choking episodes. Tragically a number of children die because the oval or rounded shape can completely block the airway. An irregular shaped object, which can still be life threatening, rarely completely obstructs the airway and usually allows some air to pass. The complicated swallowing neuromuscular coordination can also be affected by neurological disorders, stroke, surgery or other conditions, which may increase the risk of aspiration. Once swallowed, the food bolus is propelled down the esophagus by coordinated snakelike muscular action called peristalsis. It is not recommended, but peristalsis is powerful enough that you can swallow against gravity while standing on your head.

The muscular valve at the junction of the esophagus and stomach is called the lower esophageal sphincter. The lower esophageal sphincter is designed to allow food and fluid to enter the stomach, with the door closed behind them once they leave the esophagus. If the valve opens at the wrong time, gastric acid, digestive enzymes, and food can flow back into the esophagus. This can lead to symptoms of heartburn or mucosal damage. If it occurs frequently gastroesophageal reflux disease (GERD) can predispose to a change in the tissue lining of the esophagus. The growth of intestinal type tissue is called a Barrett esophagus, and is at a higher risk of cancer development than the normal tissue lining.

The stomach is a churning cauldron of muscular mixing contractions, concentrated acid secretion, and potent digestive enzymes. The vagus nerve and gut hormones play a key role in the intricate balance of enzymes, acid, nutrients, and motility. When the conditions are right, the pyloric sphincter of the stomach opens to allow the acid, enzyme, and food mixture to exit. This digestive material is now called chyme as it enters the first portion of the small intestine, known as the duodenum. In Greek, this means the width equivalent to twelve fingers, which is what its small size would measure using your digits. For its small size, the duodenum plays an amazing and complex part.

The highly acid chyme would quickly damage the lining of the duodenum if it did not respond quickly with the pouring on, much like a fire extinguisher, of sodium bicarbonate. The sodium bicarbonate is produced in the duodenum itself, as well as the pancreas. The sodium bicarbonate produced in the pancreas is released through the pancreatic duct, which empties into the duodenum through the ampulla of Vater. The fire extinguisher analogy shares another aspect of the story. Perhaps you made a fire extinguisher in a science class, or home experiment, by adding baking soda that contains sodium bicarbonate and vinegar that contains acetic acid. The active bubbling reaction that takes places is the release of carbon dioxide and water as the acid neutralizes the base. This is the same type of reaction that takes place in the duodenum, when the hydrochloric acid of the stomach meets the sodium bicarbonate released to neutralize it.

When the two react they produce water, sodium chloride commonly known as salt, and large quantities of carbon dioxide. The carbon dioxide is released as large volumes of gas that appears as a bubbles arising from the reaction. The carbon dioxide is used as the active ingredient in the fire extinguisher in the science experiment since it is heavier than air, and disrupts the oxygen supply that fire requires. In the human duodenum the carbon dioxide gas generated as a side product of acid neutralization leads to bloat and distension of the gut. The body is remarkably efficient in reducing the bloat fairly quickly, in that it absorbs the carbon dioxide into the bloodstream where it travels to the lungs to be exhaled.

The bile ducts from the liver join the duct from the pancreas bringing digestive enzymes and bicarbonate that enter the duodenum through the ampulla of Vater. Within the ampulla lies the muscular sphincter of Oddi. The name sounds like a character from the story of *The Wizard of Oz*, and that would be an appropriate analogy. The coordinated release of hormones, enzymes, muscular motility, and vagus nerve input are nothing short of wizardry in action. Subconsciously, your body can sense exactly what nutrients you have ingested. It responds by releasing the right recipe of enzymes, acid in the stomach, and bicarbonate in the duodenum, adjusting the pH as necessary. It adds just the correct amount of bile to the mix, controls the timing and volume of stomach emptying, and controls the speed of transit and intensity of mixing contractions through the length of the intestinal tract. The majority of the sensing and control feedback takes place in a small confined space the width of twelve fingers, the duodenum.

The breakdown products of the digestive process are absorbed through a sea of finger like projections called the villi. It looks like a field of waving wheat stalks, each upstanding villus is ready to use its enzymes and absorptive capacity to absorb nutrients. If you looked under the microscope you would find that each villus has thousands of even smaller villi on its surface, given the appropriate name of microvilli. All of these folds of absorptive tissue, if flattened out, would provide the equivalent absorptive capacity of a championship tennis court. This long tunnel of eagerly awaiting absorptive villi is about twenty feet long, and it is an amazingly efficient system of digestion and absorption.

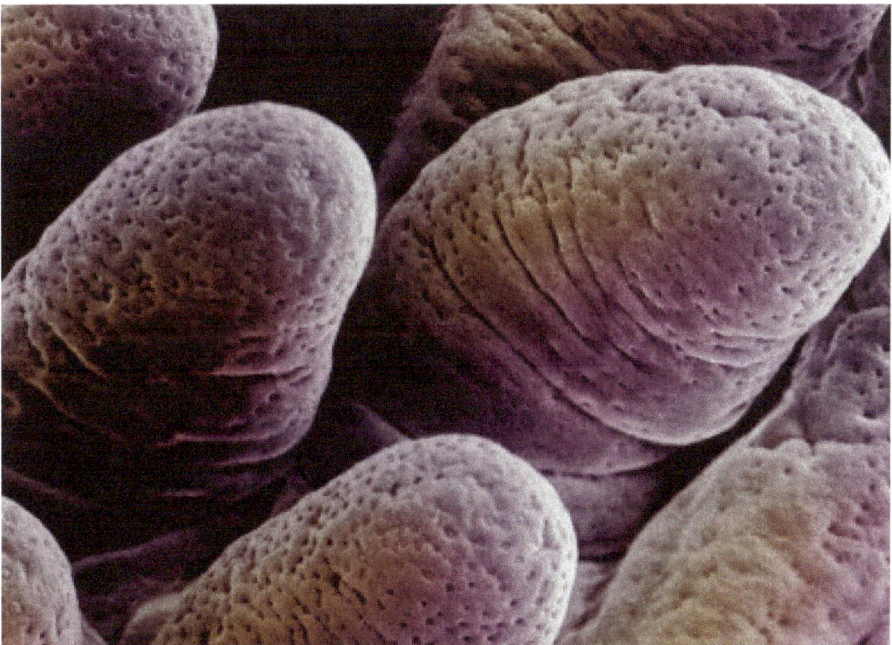

Villi in ileum of small intestine

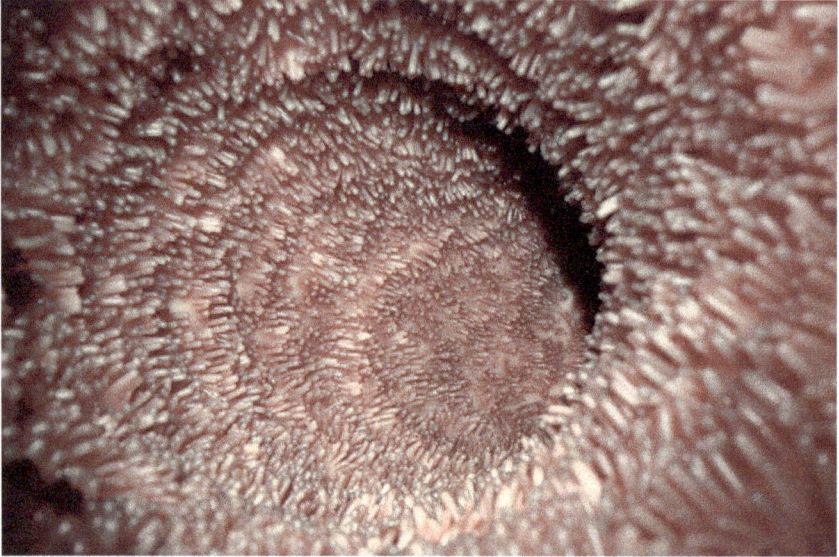

If injured, the ability of the small bowel to digest and absorb nutrients is compromised. A condition that temporarily damages the small intestine, such as a viral or bacterial gastroenteritis often called a stomach flu, can cause a blunting or shortening of the villi. The villus blunting will also lead to the loss of digestive enzymes that reside on the villi. A condition known as celiac disease (also known as gluten sensitive enteropathy, celiac sprue, non-tropical sprue, or sprue) is characterized by gluten induced damage to the villi resulting in blunting and impaired absorption of nutrients. Without the ability to digest and absorb nutrients, the unabsorbed material can cause what is known as an osmotic diarrhea. This is one of the reasons people are often advised to avoid dairy products for a week or so after stomach flu to allow the villi and enzymes to recover. If you eat or drink lactose without waiting until the recovery is complete, you may end up with symptoms of temporary lactose intolerance such as gas and diarrhea.

When the liquid chyme leaves the jejunum and ileum of the

small intestine, it goes through the ileocecal valve to enter the colon. In the cecum of the colon lies the infamous appendix, which for thousands of years mystified science as to its purpose. It looks like its function has finally, and only very recently, been identified. It stores a reservoir of intestinal bacteria, representing the healthy gut microbiome, from which the gut flora can be replenished after a bout of intestinal dysentery. The gut microbiome is much more important than most people give it credit for. The microbes of the body far outnumber the number of human cells. In fact, if you simply go by the number of cells and not their mass, they outnumber human cells by ten to one. If you look at the proportion of genes in this unified living system, over ninety-nine percent of the genes are from microbes, and only one percent is human. In other words, you as a living system are only a fraction human, and the vast majority microbes!

The majority of the microbes living within and on us are commensals. This means that they are engaged with us in a symbiotic relationship from which we both benefit. They are able to process foods that would otherwise be indigestible, and convert them to absorbable nutrients and metabolites. It is not an understatement to say that they are a requirement for our health and well-being. The gut microbiome also plays a very important role in the gut-brain-microbiome-food axis, which provides for the communication of important information between its four components. The colon, unlike the small intestine, is less involved in the digestion of foods and nutrients. It is primarily involved in the absorption of water and sodium as well as some fat-soluble vitamins such as vitamin K. The colon removes the excess moisture from the watery chyme, and the stool solidifies as it transits the gut. The ability to conserve water is very important, and without this ability the risk of dehydration would be substantially increased. The feces (also called stool, excrement, shit, and other euphemisms listed in Appendix B) is stored in the rectum and sigmoid colon awaiting the right opportunity to be eliminated through defecation.

A process or illness that impairs the colon's absorption of water will lead to more fluid in the stool and diarrhea. The loss of water and electrolytes in diarrhea may lead to dehydration, which unfortunately remains a life threatening condition in many parts of the world, especially for infants and children. If the elimination is delayed, the moisture continues to be absorbed and the stools can become harder resulting in constipation. Constipation itself aggravates the condition as the feces become harder and more difficult to pass the longer they remain in the colon. The more common treatments for constipation attempts to increase the moisture content of the feces. The feces excreted can provide information about bowel health. For most people going about their daily activities, the passage of the feces itself is the end of the story of digestion. For other organisms, including the common housefly and dung beetle, the feces are a source of nutrition. For them the elimination of feces is just the beginning of their story of digestion, and can play an important role in the transmission of disease back to humans.

Chapter Five

The Scoop on Poop

Feces (Latin fæx "dregs") are the excreted waste product from the digestive tract expelled through the anus during defecation. Although the digestive tract has extracted nutrients, the fecal matter often has fifty percent of its energy value remaining. This is a vital resource for organisms such as bacteria, fungi, and insects such as the fly and dung beetle. Human fecal matter varies significantly in appearance, depending on diet and health. A sticky gummy texture is often noted with substantial internal bleeding, which also often presents as black tarry stool called melena.

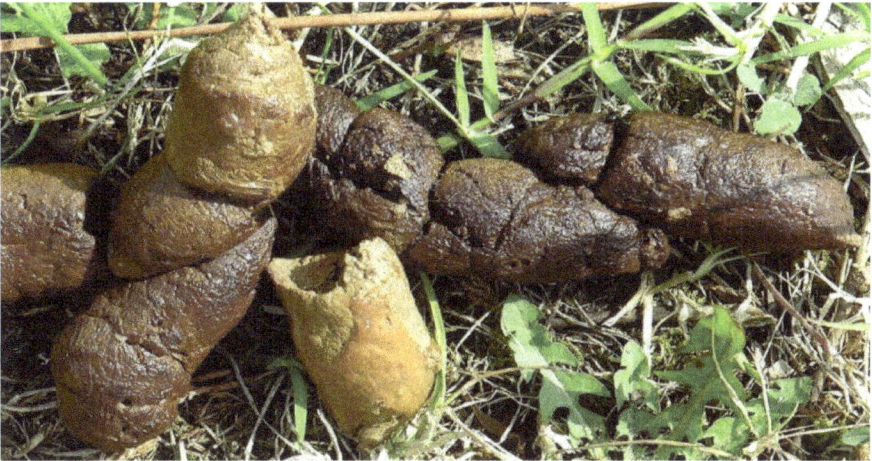

Feces on grass. Curezone.com

Brown Stool - Human feces ordinarily have a light to dark brown coloration, which results from a combination of bile and bilirubin that is derived from the breakdown products of dead red blood cells.

Yellow Stool - Stool that is yellow may suggest presence of undigested fat in the stool. The stool containing the undigested fat may appear yellowish in color, greasy, and also may smell foul. Yellowing of feces may also be caused by an infection that may also cause diarrhea, such as from *Giardia lamblia*, a protozoan parasite.

Black Stool (Melena) - Feces can be black due to the presence of red blood cells that have been broken down by digestive enzymes. This is known as melena, and is typically due to bleeding in the upper digestive tract, such as from a bleeding peptic ulcer. The same color change can be observed after consuming foods that contain a substantial proportion of animal blood, such as black pudding or tiết canh.

Black feces can also be caused by a number of medications containing bismuth products (such as Pepto-Bismol and the newer formulation of Kaopectate in the United States), iron supplements, or foods such as beetroot, black licorice, or blueberries.

Red Stool - Hematochezia is similarly the passage of feces that are bright red due to the presence of undigested blood, either from lower in the digestive tract, or from a more active source in the upper digestive tract. Ingestion of red beets will also color the stool and can be easily misinterpreted as a sign of internal bleeding. Besides the dramatic blood red color of beets, a similar red color may also come from natural or artificial coloring such as red gelatin, popsicles, Kool-Aid, and dragon fruit

Blue Stool - Prussian blue, used in the treatment of radiation, cesium, and thallium poisoning, can turn the feces blue. Substantial consumption of products containing blue food dye, such as blue curaçao or grape soda, can have a similar effect.

White (Acholic) Stool - Acholic stools, which are pasty white in color, are characteristic of complete biliary obstruction.

Silver Stool - Silver or aluminum feces color results when biliary obstruction of any type (acholic or white stool) combines with gastrointestinal bleeding from any source that would normally present as black stools or melena.

Green Stool - Feces can be green due to having large amounts of unprocessed bile in the digestive tract. When stool passes through the intestines rapidly (diarrhea) there may be little time for bilirubin to undergo its usual chemical changes. Green feces may occasionally be the result from eating liquorice candy, as it is typically made with anise oil rather than liquorice herb and is predominantly sugar. Excessive sugar consumption or a sensitivity to anise oil may cause loose, green stools.

Medical students are taught the significance of stool color. A pediatric colleague, Richard Buchta, shared the story of a professor quizzing medical students about the significance of different colored stools. The group was asked what question they should ask if a young lady told them she was passing golden stools. A witty medical student quickly responded that the question to be asked was 'Will you marry me?'

Feces are often used as fertilizer, both manure and guano becoming large commercial enterprises. Historically human waste, euphemistically called night soil, was used as a major source of fertilizer. Animal feces, especially those of camel, bison, oxen, yak, water buffalo, and cattle can be used as fuel or building material when dried. Terms such as dung, scat, spoor, manure, castings, spraint, fewmets, guano, and droppings are used to refer to specific animal feces.

Common animal dropping names are:

bat: guano	fox: billitting
cattle: tath	vermin: fuants
otter: spraints	hawk: mutes
seafowl: guano	pinniped: guano
earthworm: wormcast	dogs: scumber
dinosaur: coprolite	hare: crotiles, crotisings
hart and deer: fewmets	boar, bear, and wolf: lesses
cow: bodewash, cowpies, buffalo chips	

It is only relatively recently that science has become very

interested in poop, and the important role it can play in health as well as disease as part of the human microbiome. The microbiome is the world of microorganisms, too small to be seen with the naked eye, that exist in our environment, as well as on, in, and within our body tissue. The fact that we are surrounded by and immersed in a world of microbes has been known for a long time. What is new and surprising is the revelation that we are much more interdependent with the microbiome than science and medicine ever knew or believed.

The most remarkable finding is that the human body and its microbiome are in nearly constant communication with each other. It would not be an overstatement to describe these discoveries as revolutionary, and our understanding of health and disease is being dramatically altered. In fact, even how we consider what it means to be human, and the nature of our body, is being revised and redefined. But before we explore our relationship with the microbiome in detail, let's get some more background information, and start by taking a closer look at where microbes are within the remarkable evolutionary diversity of life on our planet Earth.

The forms of life on the planet range from the simplest organisms of a single cell or less, to multicellular organisms of increasing complexity and size. There are also a variety of major life forms that were previously classified as Kingdoms, ranging from the commonly known plants, animals, fungi, bacteria, viruses, and protozoans. Over the last few decades scientific advances have also identified new life forms including the controversial prions that are the cause of exotic diseases such as mad-cow disease (Bovine Spongiform Encephalopathy) and kuru. Even more surprising has been the discovery of a new life form called Archaea (Latin for 'ancient one'). The reason this was such an unexpected discovery is that they are in fact commonplace, and thrive in places where life was not even thought possible.

One of the reasons they were not recognized, even though

found in abundance, was that their external appearance is similar to bacteria. It was only with the advent of genomic sequencing that it was recognized that Archaea were not just a little bit different than bacteria, but so totally different that it appears as if they came from an alien planet. As strange as that thought might sound, there is a field of science called astrobiology that theorizes that that is exactly what happened. Archaea live and thrive within fuming volcanic vents, boiling hot springs, even deep inside of rocks mined miles underground. They have been transported to outer space and lived and thrived when left exposed to the unearthly vacuum outside of the space station. Because they survive and thrive in extreme environments, they have been designated as extremophiles (Latin -loving extremes).

As you may recall from the theory of evolution, developed by Charles Darwin and others, life began on the planet Earth from the simplest of organisms, to single and then multicellular organisms of increasing complexity. From submicroscopic viruses and prions that can only be visualized with extraordinarily powerful electron microscopes to enormous individual plants and fungi that stretch for miles, the abundance of life diversity on the planet is astounding. According to evolutionary theory all living things on the planet are distant relatives, all arising as the progeny of the very first single organism.

Even if you restrict your consideration to life forms that are visible to us, the diversity of appearance and activities is staggering. Humans as a species are very sensitive to physical appearance, both as a social as well as a biological consideration. Numerous studies show that our preferences for mate selection are highly driven by physical appearance. This is partly based on appearance correlating to physical and mental health, and the ability to provide support and protection. Although we have great variability in skin, hair, eye, nose, ears, height, weight, etcetera, we are virtually the same genetically. Even one of our closest evolutionary relatives, the chimpanzee, has ninety-nine percent genetic similarity to humans.

Humans are one of the largest animals in physical size. Of course we are relatively small compared to blue whales and elephants, but compared to a mouse or ants we are gigantic. There's an even more heavily populated much smaller world, invisible to the naked eye, which contains microbes. Seen by humans only with the assistance of a microscope, their invisible individual presence has a profound effect on our health and wellness. Its ability to overwhelm an organism many times its size is partly due to its rapid rate of reproduction.

The population pattern displayed by microbes, as well as other cells, is known as exponential or logarithmic growth. One cell divides and become two cells, the two cells divide and become four, the four become eight, and so forth. The power of exponential growth is often underestimated. A side story of the development of the game of chess will serve as an excellent demonstration. When the inventor of the game presented it to his King as a gift hundreds of years ago, the king was so grateful for the gift that he asked the inventor what he would like in return. The inventor asked the king for one grain of rice to be awarded him for the first square of the chessboard, two grains of rice for the second square, and each subsequent square to be given twice the amount of rice awarded for the square before. There are sixty-four squares on the chessboard and the sequence of doubling would begin with the series of numbers 1, 2, 4, 8, 16, 32, 64, 128, 256, 512, etcetera.

After the first ten squares had been added up that was less than one thousand grains of rice, and the King said he would grant him what he requested, and he was surprised that the inventor was not so smart after all and asked for such a small reward. What the King did not recognize about the power of exponential growth bankrupted his kingdom. By the time the numbers had finished doubling on the sixty-fourth square the king owed the inventor eighteen quintillion grains of rice, a number with eighteen zeros, 18,000,000,000,000,000,000! The rice would have covered the entire continents of Asia and Europe, and there was not that much rice in the entire world.

Although they are diminutive in size, microbes are metabolically active and their impact is magnified because of their enormous populations. The entire human population of the Earth is under eight billion. If you pick up a handful of soil you pick up an entire world with more microbes than the earthly human population. You have also given those microbes an experience of an earthquake of astronomical proportions! Now put them down gently, and savor an instance of power that few mortals have ever experienced and appreciated.

It should not surprise you that your skin has microbes on it; after all it is exposed to the external environment. What might surprise you are the variety and population numbers of microbes that consider your skin home. When the microbes on or in the body have established themselves as residents they are considered the microbiome, the microbial populations in that environment. If you have not heard of the term microbiome before, please add it to your vocabulary now; you will be hearing a lot more about it over the years to come.

The skin microbiome is just one of the many microbiomes of the body, and one of the most accessible. When you bathe, shower, or wash your hands you remove many of these microbes, but a sizable population remain and has made you their permanent home. Don't be upset with them however, as they are actually providing you with a valuable service in exchange for your hospitality. The vast majorities of microbes are actually beneficial to humans, and live with us in a relationship described in biological terms as symbiotic when they provide a benefit, and commensal when they do not provide a benefit but at the same time do no harm. When microbes go badly in their guest relationship with humans we describe them as pathogens. Just like plants, where the majority of plants are beneficial or do no harm, and there are just a few harmful ones like poison ivy, the microbial pathogens are very few in number.

The skin has different features and characteristics dependent on body location, and the microbiome is unique to each area as well. Various skin products including soaps with anti-microbial activity, lotions, massage oils, as well as swimming, bathing, clothing, and other environmental factors can influence the skin microbiome. In Ayurveda the various oils and botanicals applied in massage and skin therapy undoubtedly effect the skin microbiome.

What many people find surprising is that the intestinal tract, normally considered an internal organ, is actually an external organ just like the skin, as far as the body is concerned. The reason for this 'inside out' logic is that the external environment continues all the way through the gut, from mouth to anus. The material within the digestive tract is considered outside of the body until it is absorbed through the intestinal lining. Because this is a potential source of infection and allergies, the body has a powerful and vigilant immune system that is extremely active in the gut.

As you can imagine, a lot of microbes live in the mouth, between the teeth, under the gums, in the nasal passages, etcetera. A large number of microbes entered your mouth on the surface or within the food you ate, joining with the microbes who have already established this part of your body as their permanent home. These microbes are feasting on small particles of food and debris left over from the chewing process, even when you brush and floss well.

The microbes in the mouth and within the food are regularly swallowed and travel down the digestive tract on an amazing voyage that would make any theme park ride pale in comparison. For many of the bacteria this is a nightmare journey at the ends of their lives, and for others it is the equivalent of being transported to heaven. The microbes making this journey contribute to the gut microbiome, which is the largest microbiome of the body, numbering over one-hundred trillion organisms. This astronomical number is greater than the number of stars in the universe, and collectively weighs in at about three pounds.

Measured by cell populations the average human is ten percent human cells and ninety percent microbial cells. If you look at a more important factor, gene activity, the human genome has about twenty-five thousand genes, and the microbiome well in excess of one million, making us only one percent human genes. The gut microbiome is much more than just fermenting or metabolizing food products our own intestinal tract cannot digest. Amazingly, the gut microbiome engages in an active two-way communication with the human brain, and through epigenetics with every aspect of the human experience.

Communication is one of the hallmarks of higher animals, and language has traditionally been thought to be a uniquely human trait. Science is exploring the communication of other animals and it appears that they also use language of a limited vocabulary that is primarily used to warn of danger. More research is ongoing into the modes of communication of other animals, from the vocalization of whales that communicate over distances of many miles at sea, to the recently discovered elephant communication at extremely low frequency below the range of human hearing.

Now don't get too disappointed as I am not going to surprise you and tell you that the microbes speak to you in quiet internal voices, the microbial whisperers. Besides, you already know that humans and other species frequently communicate, as we do routinely with pets. This is especially clear when cats command their human servants to feed them. From dog whisperers and trainers, to the simple dog facial expressions of joy and remorse, nonverbal communication is a regular occurrence. Even plants communicate with each other, often through the air by releasing volatile chemical messengers warning of pathogens and danger. In the case of the microbiome, the communication takes place in the common language of most living organisms, chemical neurotransmitters, hormones, and metabolites. This is a language the microbes, body, and brain instantly recognize and understand.

The gut microbiome weighs in at about three pounds, roughly the same weight as the human brain, and interestingly enough, is part of what is now commonly known as the 'second brain' comprised of the gut-microbiome-brain axis. This 'second brain' is adding a scientific understanding to what has commonly been described as gut feelings or gut instincts. The subject is fascinating, and is covered in greater detail in other books in this series described in the afterword.

Chapter Six

Tushy Hygiene

Anal cleansing after defecation was historically accomplished with sticks, leaves, stones, clay, corncobs, water, or literally whatever was available at hand. The ancient Greeks used clay and stone. Romans used a water soaked sponge on a stick. Toilet paper has been used for the cleaning of the anus and urethra after elimination for well over one thousand years. The first recorded use of toilet paper was in China in the sixth century.

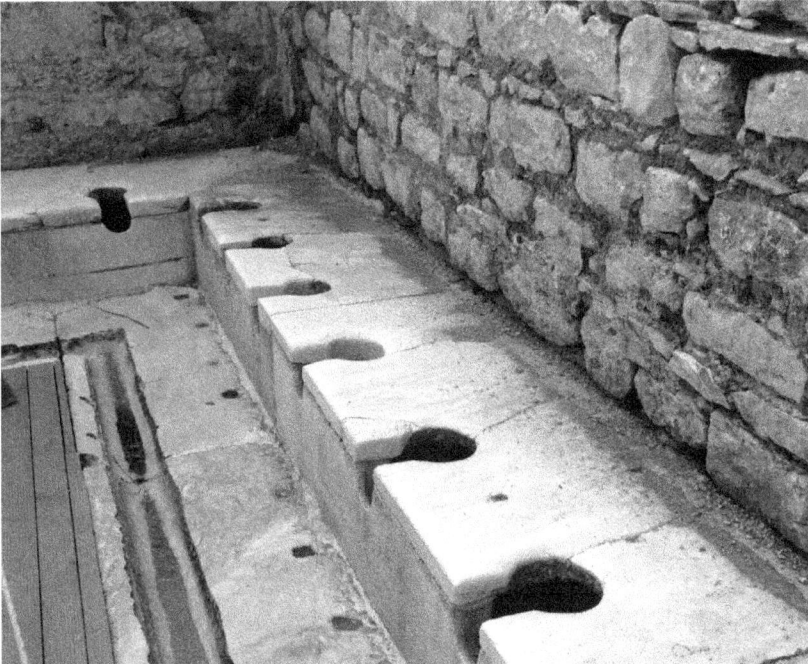

Ancient Roman latrines in Ostia Antica. Toilets in ancient Rome had sophisticated sewer lines with running water to remove waste. Remarkably many countries around the world have more primitive systems in place today than the Romans had over two thousand years ago.
Shutterstock/AbelFeyman

Toilet is derived from the French word toilette meaning the act of washing, dressing, and preparing oneself. In Western society human feces waste management is usually a matter of a toilet with indoor plumbing, and a sewer or septic system. Anal cleansing after defecation was historically accomplished with sticks, leaves, stones, clay, corncobs, water, or literally whatever was available at hand. In many parts of the world only the left hand was used for wiping and cleansing after defecation. That may have contributed to the use of the right hand for social greetings and shaking hands.

The Hongwu Emperor was the first ruler of the Ming dynasty (1368-1644). Chinese imperial court documents show that fifteen thousand sheets of 'thick but soft' perfumed toilet paper were ordered in 1393. The royal family was recorded as using 720,000 sheets of toilet paper a year. The large sheets of two feet by three feet were for general use at the court, but smaller and even better quality sheets that were three inches square were designed for the exclusive use of the imperial family.

In the United States toilet paper was often simply pages torn out of the Farmer's Almanac, or the catalog of merchants such as Sears, Roebuck. & Company. They often came with a pre-punched hole in the catalog for ease of hanging by wire in the bathroom or outhouse. A humorous spinoff on the Sears Roebuck catalog was the 'Rears and Sorebutt' catalog. New York entrepreneur Joseph Gayetty invented aloe-infused sheets of Manila hemp in 1857 that he claimed prevented hemorrhoids. The product was sold in 500 sheet packages and marketed as Gayetty's Medicated Paper. The name Gayetty was imprinted on each sheet of the patented paper, and he was happy to see his name so besmirched as his fortune increased every time his customers wiped.

In 1872 John Kimberly, Charles Clark, and other investors started a paper manufacturing company in Wisconsin. In 1874 the brothers Thomas, Clarence, and E. Irvin Scott created a competing paper company and in 1890 popularized toilet paper on a roll. Scott advertised that "over 65% of middle-aged men and women suffered from some sort of rectal disease".

The Scott brothers claimed that inferior toilet paper was responsible and that "harsh toilet tissue may cause serious injury". The advertisement went on to say "ScotTissue, Sani-tissue and Waldorf are famous bathroom tissues specifically processed to satisfy the three requirements doctors say toilet tissue must have to be safe: absorbency-softness-chemical purity".

In 1901 the Northern Paper Mills in Green Bay Wisconsin developed a toilet paper that was not made from hardwood pulp, but from softer pulp. They advertised it as the first toilet tissue that guaranteed you would not get wood splinters on wiping. The appeal of not getting wood splinters on wiping with toilet paper not surprisingly led to immediate market success. Competitors soon joined in the rush to market splinter free toilet paper.

By 1925 the Scott brothers were the largest toilet paper manufacturers in the world. Acquired by Kimberly-Clark in 1995 for just under ten billion US dollars, the Scott brand name of toilet paper remains very popular. Twenty-six billion rolls of toilet paper are sold annually in the United States. Americans use an average of twenty-three and a half rolls per capita a year.

One tree produces about one hundred pounds (forty-five kilograms) of toilet paper, and global production consumes twenty-seven thousand trees daily. Perforated toilet paper for ease of tearing off sheets was patented in 1871 by New York businessman Seth Wheeler. He established the Albany Perforated Wrapping Paper Company, and toilet paper in those days was more politely referred to as wrapping paper. The patent application specified that the end of the roll of toilet paper was to be on the outside or in the 'over' position. Although the subject of ongoing debate, controversy, and arguments within a household, the official patented invention specifies 'over', and seventy percent of the public dutifully complies.

The toilet paper business in the United States is an enormous enterprise. The industry is innovative in finding ways to increase profit margins. According to the financial newspaper The Wall Street Journal in 2013 the Kimberley-Clark Corporation announced that it improved its toilet paper product by making it fifteen percent bulkier, but at the same time reduced the number of sheets by thirteen percent, a process the industry terms desheeting. Desheeting while making bulkier tissue is a money saver as Kimberly-Clark says it doesn't need additional material to make its sheets fluffier. Kimberly Clark is the largest manufacturer of toilet paper in the world with products sold in over 150 countries.

Toilet Paper was medicated, perforated, perfumed, and considered the state the art of anal hygiene in the mid-nineteenth century. Creative Commons License

According to Kimberly-Clark's research, Americans use on average forty-six sheets of toilet paper a day over five bathroom trips. Over eighty-three million rolls of toilet paper are manufactured in the United States each day. In 2012 companies sold over ten billion dollars of tissue and toilet paper, a two percent increase over the previous year. Seven billion rolls of toilet paper are sold each year in the United States. In the U.S. more than fifty miles of toilet paper are produced every second. A roll of toilet paper will last five days in the average U.S. household. The average American uses one hundred rolls of toilet paper (twenty thousand sheets) per year, and will require the processing of 384 trees during their lifetime to create the toilet paper they will use.

Most of the world has embraced the use of water cleansing for hygienic purposes wherever available. Approximately four billion people around the world do not use toilet paper. The use of only paper products for anal hygiene is counterintuitive, and is surprisingly still the procedure of choice in the United States and many Western countries. The last figures for toilet paper consumption by country were published over twenty years ago. The US led the world with 730 pounds of toilet paper consumption per resident each year. Other countries on the list with pounds of consumption per year for each resident included Finland 669, Belgium 565, Japan 526, Canada 505, Singapore 502, Taiwan 492, Switzerland 476, Denmark 471, New Zealand 468, Brazil 77, China 48, Indonesia 31, and Russia 28. Since the list was published Japan has moved into second place and China a rapidly rising third place.

Designer toiler papers are very popular. They come in various colors, but white remain the most popular followed by beige, and peach. Some come with embossed patterns, and others with writings, poetry, and images. The most exclusive designer toilet paper comes from Japan, where the Hanebisho Company creates handcrafted toilet paper that sells for nearly $20 per roll. It is created from the highest quality wood fiber pulp from

Canada, and treated with the purest water fin Japan from the Nyodo River. The special drying process is constantly adjusted for humidity and temperature. The paper is then decorated by highly trained artisans and carefully wrapped and packaged in special decorative boxes. The product has been delivered to the residence of the Emperor of Japan for years.

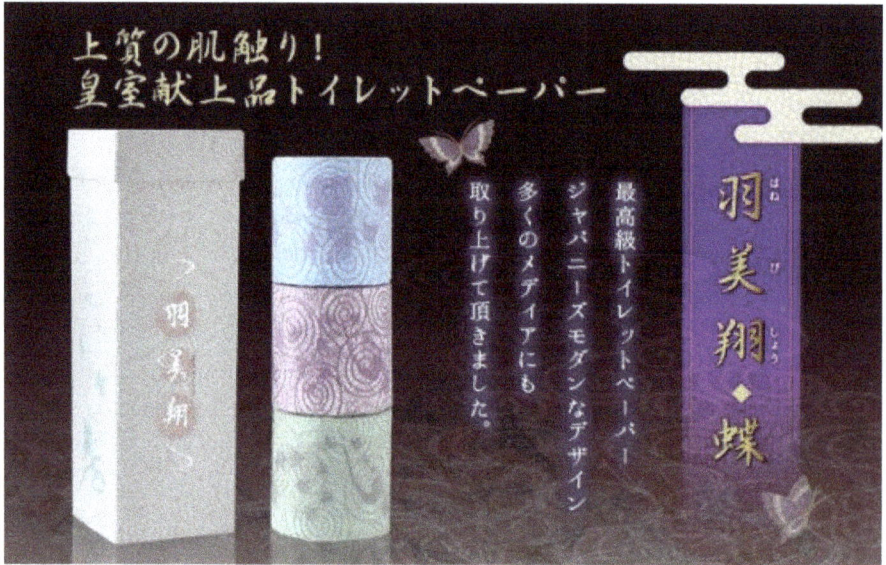

If you were to take toilet paper in your bare hands to wipe your pet or child's behind after a bowel movement, you would probably instantly recognize the unhygienic nature of the activity and wash your hands thoroughly. If you did not know it before now you do, toilet paper has to be at least ten sheets thick to prevent bacteria from easily transiting through the porous paper. Even double and triple folding of toilet paper allows fecal bacteria to be in direct contact with the hands. After wiping the person touches the handle to flush. It should not come as any surprise that the toilet faucet or handle has four hundred times the number of bacteria per square inch than the toilet seat.

In the United States and Western society many people wipe after a bowel movement with only porous toilet tissue paper between their fingers and fecal material. These same fingers are then often used to prepare food or pick up finger food that is often shared with others. In the United States health department codes require that restaurant and food preparation employees wash their hands after using the bathroom. The best approach is to practice regular hand washing with an anti-microbial soap and water. The lack of hand washing after using the bathroom is commonplace, as is the lack of basic hand washing skills. The use of an ultraviolet backlight below demonstrates how the hands harbor pockets of potential sources of infection. The touching of a toilet handle and door knob on leaving the bathroom can allow the further transmission of infectious microbes.

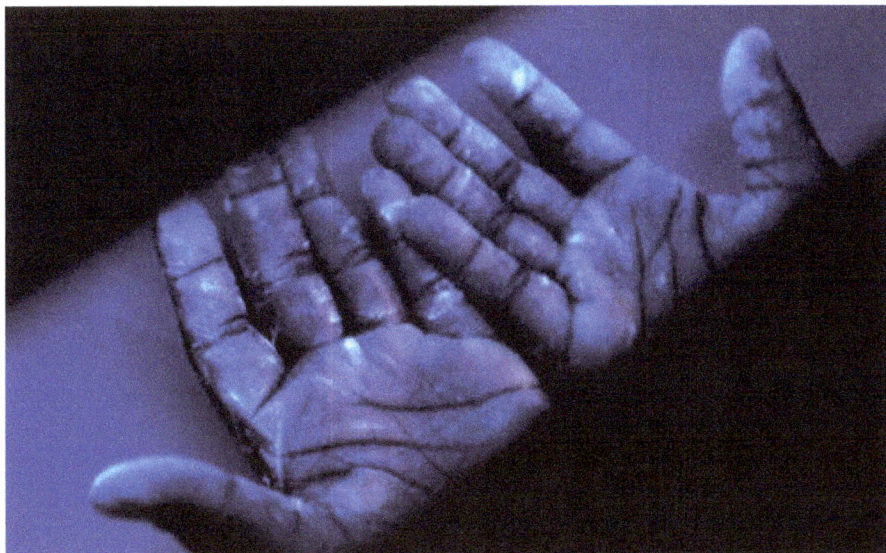

OUTFOXprevention.com. Used with Permission.

The United States Center for Disease Control publishes the following guidelines for proper hand washing. Wet the hands with clean, running water (warm or cold), turn off the tap, and apply soap. Lather the hands by rubbing them together with the soap. Lather the backs of hands, between fingers, and under the nails. Scrub the hands for at least twenty seconds. Rinse the hands well under clean, running water. Dry the hands using a clean towel or air-dry them.

The U.S. CDC advocates washing hands before, during, and after preparing food, before eating food, before and after caring for someone who is sick, before and after treating a cut or wound, after using the toilet, and after changing diapers or cleaning up a child who has used the toilet. Hand washing is also recommended after nose blowing, coughing, or sneezing, after touching an animal, animal feed, or animal waste, after handling pet food or pet treats, and after touching garbage.

Alcohol based hand sanitizers that contain at least sixty percent ethanol is also effective in reducing the transmission of contaminants and infective agents. Hopefully, the advent of high technology toilets incorporating automatic water washing features, as well as warm air blow-drying, obviating the need for toilet paper and touching the anogenital area will be more readily embraced by Western and other cultures. Contrary to popular belief Thomas Crapper did not invent the indoor flush toilet. It had been developed hundreds of years before he established his manufacturing company in Victorian England.

Credit for the flushing toilet is usually attributed to Sir John Harrington, a godson of Queen Elizabeth I. One rumor is that his first name is the source of the nickname 'john' for a toilet. Thomas Crapper had a successful plumbing business and the inventor Albert Giblin was an employee of his. Giblin patented a silent siphon valve and Crapper bought the patent and marketed the improved toilet from 1861-1904 at great profit and name recognition.

The average person goes to the toilet 2,500 times per year, and spends a total of three years of their lifetime sitting on the toilet. For those musically inclined most toilets flush in the key of E flat. Other trivia of note, one third of Americans flush the toilet while still sitting on it, and there are 40,000 injuries a year while sitting on the toilet seat. In France the invention of the bidet in the early eighteenth century made water cleansing popular. The word bidet means pony in French, and using the bidet required that one straddle the bowl of the bidet as if riding a pony.

A bidet spray or health faucet is a hand held hose and nozzle that utilizes a water spray for perianal and genitourinary cleansing after defecation and urination. The bidet is commonplace in many countries including Spain (thirty percent), Portugal (seventy percent), Greece (eighty percent), Italy (ninety-five percent), and Japan (fifty percent). In Japan automated and high technology toilets incorporate water washing as well as air blow drying and other features. The water bidet is also very popular in the Middle East, and growing in popularity in the United States.

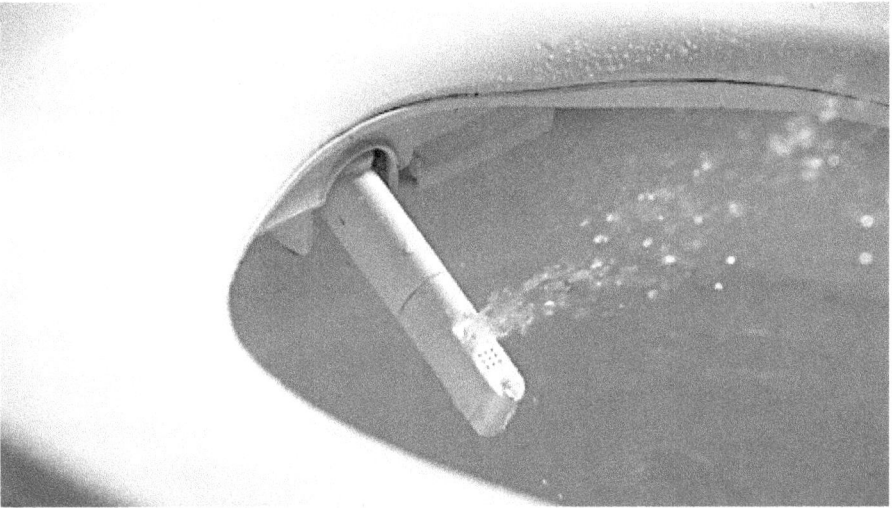

Although popular in Europe and elsewhere around the world, the United States has been very slow to adopt the preferable water based approach to anal hygiene. In addition to its increased efficacy it has environmental benefits in reducing forest product consumption and sewage disposal of paper waste products. Creative Commons License

Although popular in Europe and elsewhere around the world, the United States has been very slow to adopt the preferable water based approach to anal hygiene. In addition to its increased efficacy it has environmental benefits in reducing forest product consumption and sewage disposal of paper waste products. The reluctance of Americans to adopt the use of the bidet may be related to a misconception on the part of American and British troops during World War I. When they were first exposed to the bidet in France they assumed its purpose was purely for the washing of the genitals after sexual intercourse. The bidet incorrectly became associated as a product developed to accommodate French sexual immorality.

Although there are some very expensive models of toilets combined with bidets, the cost of an aftermarket addition of a washlet feature to a toilet is very economical. Many bidet equivalent washlets cost less than one hundred dollars, and with the savings by reduced toilet paper usage the device rapidly pays for itself. On the Indian subcontinent, in spite of the lack of bidets, over ninety-five percent of the population use water for anal cleansing. Many also use soap with water for cleansing after defecating. Use of paper is rare in this region, and hand washing after cleansing is critically important to prevent illness.

In Japan the technological innovation of combining the bidet and toilet into a single product was introduced and advanced. Rapid innovations included a heated seat, automatic deodorizing, automatic lid raising and closing, directed water jets for female and male anatomy, music playing during use, vacuum fan ventilation, and warm air blow drying to obviate the need for wiping or use of toilet paper.

Genital and anal infections do not come in contact with the toilet seat in normal use. The intact skin of your buttocks is an efficient barrier against most disease organisms. Most transmission of pathogens is via the fecal to oral route is usually accomplished by way of the hands. The flush handle, sink handles, and door knob are much more likely to be a source of contamination since they are much likely to have been touched by someone whose hands had just been used to wipe their bottoms with a thin piece of toilet paper. It would be a good precaution to use toilet paper or paper towels to prevent your hands from touching the flush, faucet, and doorknobs or handles.

Most transmission of pathogens is via the fecal to oral route is usually accomplished by way of the hands. The average human stool contains three trillion microorganisms. Wiping with toilet paper nearly guarantees that the hands will come into contact with fecal microorganisms. After wiping it is not uncommon to find brown streaks on underwear because of inadequate anal hygiene. The average man's underwear contains one-tenth of a gram of feces at laundering.

Another infection risk from the toilet is the splashing and aerosol formation that can occur during flushing, particularly when someone with diarrhea has used that toilet. Surprisingly one-third of Americans remain seated on the toilet when they flush, and perhaps mistakenly find the misting of their anogenital region refreshing and hygienic. If they put paper toilet seat covers down before they sit on a public toilet seat for hygienic purposes, they should definitely get off the toilet seat before they flush.

The typical toilet flush creates a mist of contaminated water droplets that can travel up to twenty feet in all directions. It includes fecal matter and pathogens that settle on any exposed surface in the flush zone, including toothbrushes, drinking cups, bath toys, handles and doorknobs. The mist can stay airborne for up to two hours and be easily inhaled. The microbial pathogens can live on surfaces for up to a week. Before you flush, lower the lid to keep the aerosolization and spread to a minimum.

Worldwide there are approximately two million fatalities every year due to diarrhea. The majority of these are in children under five years of age. Simple routine hand washing with soap and water could reduce the incidence of diarrhea by approximately fifty percent, and respiratory infections by about twenty-five percent. Hand washing also reduces the incidence of skin diseases, eye infections, and intestinal worms and parasites.

Annual deaths of children under five from diarrhoea (thousands, estimated)[5]

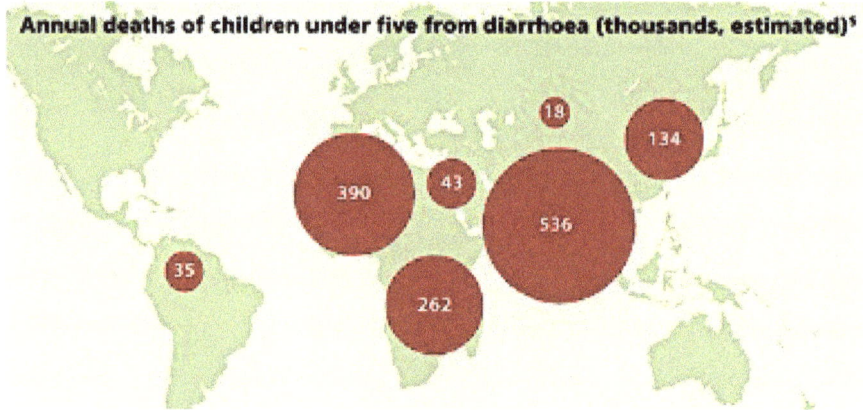

uwcm-geog.wikispaces.com/Food+Aid Creative Commons License

In most cultures and faiths food is not stored, prepared, or consumed in the vicinity of a toilet area. Both Islam and Judaism have a brief prayer of thanksgiving to be offered after the body functions of eliminating waste and the washing of hands. With the risk to health and wellness from exposure to human waste, religious customs and practices often offered practical guidance and hygiene to avoid disease.

Istinja (Arabic: استنجاء), a component of Islamic hygiene practices, is the cleansing away of any residue and impurities (najasat) that remain after being passed from the urethra or anus. Istinja requires the use of water if available, and may be utilized with water alone or in combination with toilet paper. If water is not available stones, soil, or other natural material (other than bone or dung) may be utilized in the process known as 'istijmar'. The passage of intestinal gas alone does not require Istinja

Xylospongium, also known as *sponge on a stick*, is a device used to clean the perianal area after a bowel movement. It consists of a wooden stick (Greek: ξύλον, *Xylon*) with a sponge (Greek: Σπόγγος, *Spongos*) fixed at one end. In the *baths of the seven sages* in Ostia, a fresco from the 2nd century contains the Inscription *(u)taris xylosphongio* which is the first known mention of the term. Also in the early second century a papyrus letter of Claudius Terentianus to his father Claudius Tiberianus uses the term *xylospongium* in a phrase.

Shit stick is a thin stake or stick used for cleaning the perianal area after a bowel movement. It is used when water or toilet paper was not available for this purpose. The term has also been used in Chinese Buddhism and Japanese Buddhism. A well-known example is *gānshǐjué/kanshiketsu* (乾屎橛 "dry shit stick") from the Chan/Zen *gōng'àn/kōan* in which a monk asked "What is Buddha?" and Master Yunmen/Unmon answered "A dry shit stick".

The presumed logic for such language was that most of the great masters of these schools did not directly state what they wished to convey. They often used a shout, or strike with a rod, or striking phrase as above to place their student in a state between comprehensibility and incomprehensibility. According to this logic it somehow promoted their development of enlightenment." Another explanation was that Zen Buddhist masters used the image of a dry shit stick to neutralize and balance of our image of a true person as sine thing other than pure or noble.

People have used many different materials in the long history of anal cleansing, including leaves, rags, paper, water, sponges, corncobs, earthenware, pottery, and sticks. In ancient times, instruments made from bamboo, possibly in the form of spatulas ([*cèchóu*] 廁籌, [*cèbì*] 廁箆, or [*cèjiǎn*] 廁簡), may have been used with water for cleansing after a bowel movement. the assistance of water in cleaning the body after defecation.

When monks and missionaries introduced Buddhism into China and Japan, they also brought the Indian custom of using a *śalākā, a* small stake, stick, or rod for wiping away fecal residue after a bowel movement. Translators rendered this Sanskrit word into a number of different terms based on the words *chóu* or *chū* 籌 "small stake or stick", or *jué* or *ketsu* 橛 "short stake or stick". Such teens included the Chinese *cèchóu* 廁籌 and Japanese *chūgi* 籌木. The custom of using shit sticks became popular and had the advantages of being inexpensive, washable, and reusable.

The Chinese invented paper around the 2nd century BCE, and toilet paper no later than the 6th century CE, when Yan Zhitui noted, "Paper on which there are quotations or commentaries from the Five Classics or the names of sages, I dare not use for toilet purposes". The earliest Japanese flush toilets date from the Nara period (710–784), when a drainage system was constructed in the capital at Nara. It was designed as squat toilets built over 4 - 6 inch (10–15 cm) wide wooden conduits that users would straddle. Archaeological excavations in Nara have also found numerous *chūgi* wooden sticks that were used for fecal cleansing.

The English language has some *shit(e) stick* parallels in its lexicography parallel to these Asian language terms.
The *Oxford English Dictionary* (shyte, shite, shit) quotes two early *shit-stick* examples: "a hard chuffe, a shite-sticks" (1598) and "a shite-sticks, a shite-rags, that is to say, a miserable pinch-pennie" (1659); and defines poop-stick as "a fool, ineffectual person", with the earliest usage in 1930.

Genital and anal infections do not come in contact with the toilet seat in normal use. The intact skin of your buttocks is an efficient barrier against most disease organisms. Most transmission of pathogens is via the fecal to oral route is usually accomplished by way of the hands. The average human stool contains three trillion microorganisms. Wiping with toilet paper nearly guarantees that the hands will come into contact with fecal microorganisms. After wiping it is not uncommon to find brown streaks on underwear because of inadequate anal hygiene.

The flush handle, sink handles, and door knob are much more likely to be a source of contamination since they are much likely to have been touched by someone whose hands had just been used to wipe their bottoms with a thin piece of toilet paper. It would be a good precaution to use toilet paper or paper towels to prevent your hands from touching the flush, faucet, and doorknobs or handles.

Another infection risk from the toilet is the splashing and aerosol formation that can occur during flushing, particularly when someone with diarrhea has used that toilet. Surprisingly one-third of Americans remain seated on the toilet when they flush, and perhaps mistakenly find the misting of their anogenital region refreshing and hygienic. If they put paper toilet seat covers down before they sit on a public toilet seat for hygienic purposes, they should definitely get off the toilet seat before they flush.

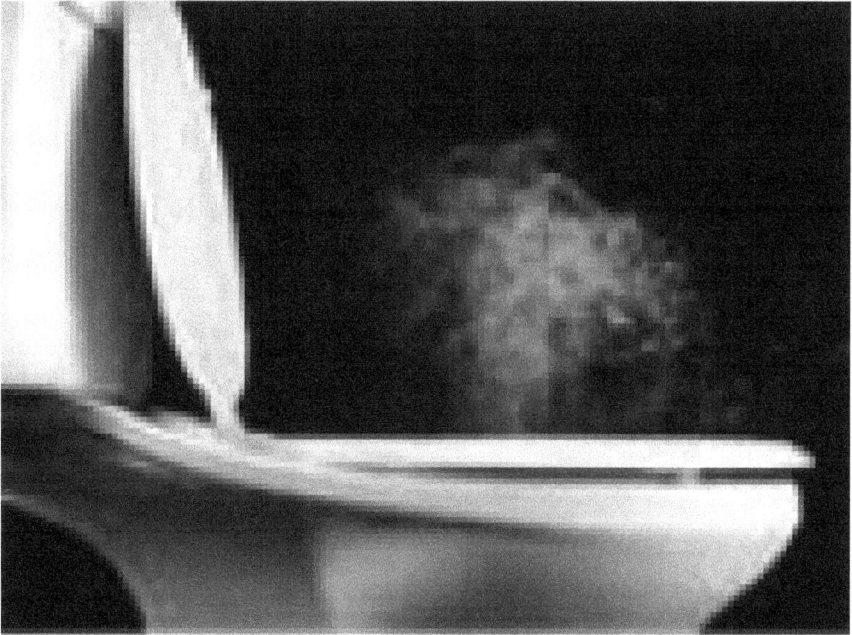

The microscopic mist that emanates with each flush of the toilet bowl distributes contaminated water droplets up to twenty feet in reach direction. Creative Commons License

The typical toilet flush creates a mist of contaminated water droplets that can travel up to twenty feet in all directions. It includes fecal matter and pathogens that settle on any exposed surface in the flush zone, including toothbrushes, drinking cups, bath toys, handles and doorknobs. The mist can stay airborne for up to two hours and be easily inhaled. The microbial pathogens can live on surfaces for up to a week. Before you flush, lower the lid to keep the aerosolization and spread to a minimum.

The best approach is to practice regular hand washing with an anti-microbial soap and water. The lack of hand washing after using the bathroom is commonplace, as is the lack of basic hand washing skills. The use of an ultraviolet backlight below demonstrates how the hands harbor pockets of potential sources of infection. The touching of a toilet handle and door knob on leaving the bathroom can allow the further transmission of infectious microbes.

Microbiological surveillance studies of *Escherichia coli* and other fecal bacteria have been performed in typical American household kitchens and bathrooms. The surprising finding was that toilet seats were one of the cleanest areas in the house with a very low microbe count. Faucets and refrigerator handles were more heavily contaminated. The highest concentration of microbes, more than two hundred times that of the toilet seat, were found on kitchen cutting boards. It was theorized this was from poultry, which often has fecal microbe contaminants in processing.

Public toilet seats were also surveyed and less than two percent had any *Escherichia coli* or fecal contaminants. Even this small percentage was thought to represent contamination from the water mist that is generated by flushing. The best use of the toilet seat paper protector dispensed would be to use it instead of your bare hands to touch the faucets and door handles in the bathroom. In other public places some of the highest concentrations of fecal bacteria are found on sanitary napkin dispensers, hotel TV remote control units, vending machine buttons, and drinking water fountain controls.

The following twenty-five locations were surveyed in the United States for fecal contaminants with some surprising findings. Fast food restaurants in the US serve ice that had more bacteria than the toilet water in seventy percent of locations surveyed. Public restrooms have about two million bacteria per square inch, while the average toilet seat has only fifty per square inch. The average office desk has four hundred times more bacteria than a toilet. Keyboards can have up to two hundred times more bacteria than a toilet seat. Cell phones and mobile electronic devices can have ten times more bacteria than a toilet seat, and they are frequently in close contact with the fingers, face, and mouth.

There are on average one hundred times more bacteria on restaurant menus than on restroom toilet seat. Raw meat carries a very high level of fecal bacteria, so food-chopping boards harbor more fecal contaminants than toilet seats. When the toilet is flushed the plume of toilet water with fecal contaminants often end up on toothbrushes left exposed. With two hundred thousand bacteria per square inch, carpets are four thousand times dirtier than a toilet seat. Humans shed one and one-half million skin cells every hour that helps feed the bacteria carpeting the carpets.

Most refrigerators test positive for the fecal contaminant *Escherichia coli* because thorough cleaning and disinfecting is an infrequent undertaking. Reusable shopping bags have more fecal matter than underwear and are rarely washed. In many households the television remote control is one of the most contaminated items handled. Hands are one of the dirtiest parts of the body, and they are frequently used to grasp and hold doorknobs, which are a reservoir of contaminants. Light switches can have up to two hundred and seventeen bacteria per square inch.

The kitchen sink is usually dirtier than the bathroom and is often overlooked when cleaning. The bathtub, although thought of as a place to get clean, typically harbors nearly twenty thousand bacteria per square inch around the drain. Dead skins cells, dust mites, fungal spores, pollens, and other body secretions build up on the pillow, the place the head usually rests at night. After ten years a mattress will nearly double in weight thanks to the number of dust mites and dust mite feces that it has collected. The inside rim of a pet bowl alone contains over two thousand bacteria per square inch.

Currency bank notes can harbor up to two hundred thousand bacteria. It's a good idea to wash the hands after directly handling cash and currency. It brings new meaning to those having lots of money being known as 'filthy rich'. Draperies collect pet fur, mold, dander, debris, dust mites, and dust mite feces. The warm, dark, and moist insides of showerheads are popular breeding grounds for bacteria. Handbags contain cell phone, money, hairbrush, lipstick, cosmetics, and other items teeming with contaminants. Handbags are rarely cleaned and are a notorious source of potential contaminants.

The kitchen sponge is nearly always the most heavily contaminated item in the house. With ten million bacteria per square inch the kitchen sponge is nearly a quarter of a million times dirtier than a toilet seat. The toilet seat is usually very clean, and the reason is really pretty simple, it gets cleaned often.

Worldwide there are approximately two million fatalities every year due to diarrhea. The majority of these are in children under five years of age. Simple routine hand washing with soap and water could reduce the incidence of diarrhea by approximately fifty percent, and respiratory infections by about twenty-five percent. Hand washing also reduces the incidence of skin diseases, eye infections, and intestinal worms and parasites.

In most cultures and faiths food is not stored, prepared, or consumed in the vicinity of a toilet area. Both Islam and

Judaism have a brief prayer of thanksgiving to be offered after the body functions of eliminating waste and the washing of hands. With the risk to health and wellness from exposure to human waste, religious customs and practices often offered practical guidance and hygiene to avoid disease.

Chapter Seven

Time to Waste, Where Does It All Go?

In Western society human feces waste management is usually a matter of indoor plumbing, a toilet, and a sewer or septic system. Animal waste, especially of dairy herds, cattle, pig farms, poultry houses, domestic pets, are a source of challenges and often commercialized solutions. Human feces waste management, especially outside of but even within Western society, is a major health and public safety concern. Although there are some very expensive models of toilets combined with bidets, the cost of an aftermarket addition of a washlet feature to a toilet is very economical. Many bidet equivalent washlets cost less than one hundred dollars, and with the savings by reduced toilet paper usage the device rapidly pays for itself.

On the Indian subcontinent, in spite of lack of bidets, over ninety-five percent of the population use water with or without soap for cleansing after defecating. Use of paper is rare in this region, and hand washing after cleansing is critically important. It is surprising that washing with water is not more universally popular as it adds another dimension of hygiene and provides an attractive and more hygienic approach than using one's hands and dry paper for anogenital cleansing. Genital and anal infections do not come in contact with the toilet seat in normal use. The intact skin of your buttocks is an efficient barrier against most disease organisms. Most transmission of pathogens is via the fecal to oral route is usually accomplished by way of the hands.

The flush handle, sink handles, and door knob are more likely to be a source of contamination since they are likely to have been touched by someone whose hands had just been used to wipe their bottoms with a flimsy piece of toilet paper. They harbor more than four-hundred times the number of bacteria per square inch as the toilet seat. It would be a good precaution to use toilet paper or paper towel as well to prevent your hands from touching the flush, faucet, and doorknobs or handles. Another infection risk from the toilet is the splashing and aerosol formation that can occur during flushing, particularly when someone with diarrhea has used the toilet. Surprisingly one third of Americans remain sitting on the toilet seat when they flush the toilet. The typical toilet flush creates a mist of contaminated water droplets that can travel up to twenty feet in all directions. It includes fecal matter and pathogens that settle on any exposed surface in the flush zone, including toothbrushes, drinking cups, bath toys, handles, and doorknobs. The mist can stay airborne for up to two hours and be easily inhaled. The microbial pathogens can live on surfaces for up to a week. Before you flush, lower the lid to keep the aerosolization and spread to a minimum.

The best approach is to practice regular hand washing with an antimicrobial soap and water. The lack of hand washing after using the bathroom is commonplace, as is the lack of basic hand washing skills. The use of an ultraviolet back light below demonstrates how the hands harbor pockets of potential sources of infection even after typical hand washing. The touching of a toilet handle and door knob on leaving the bathroom can allow the further transmission of infectious microbes. Worldwide there are approximately two million fatalities every year due to diarrhea. The majority of these are in children under five years of age. Routine hand washing with soap and water could reduce diarrhea by almost fifty percent and respiratory infections by nearly twenty-five percent. Hand washing also reduces the incidence of skin diseases, eye infections, and intestinal worms and parasites.

In most cultures and faiths food is not to be brought into or consumed in the vicinity of a toilet area. Both Islam and Judaism have a brief prayer of thanksgiving to be offered after relieving themselves, and injunctions separating such activities from the eating of food. With the risk to health and wellness from exposure to human waste the religious customs and practices offered practical guidance on hygiene to avoid disease

Feces waste management has been a concern from pre-Biblical times: "And thou shalt have a paddle upon thy weapon; and it shall be, when thou wilt ease thyself abroad, thou shalt dig therewith, and shalt turn back and cover that which cometh from thee: For the LORD thy God walketh in the midst of thy camp, to deliver thee, and to give up thine enemies before thee; therefore shall they camp be holy: that he see no unclean thing in thee, and turn away from thee." (Deuteronomy 23:13-14) Let's see how much progress human civilization has made over the thousands of years from this 'passage' from the Old Testament.

Countries with most open defecation and worst access to sanitation[3]

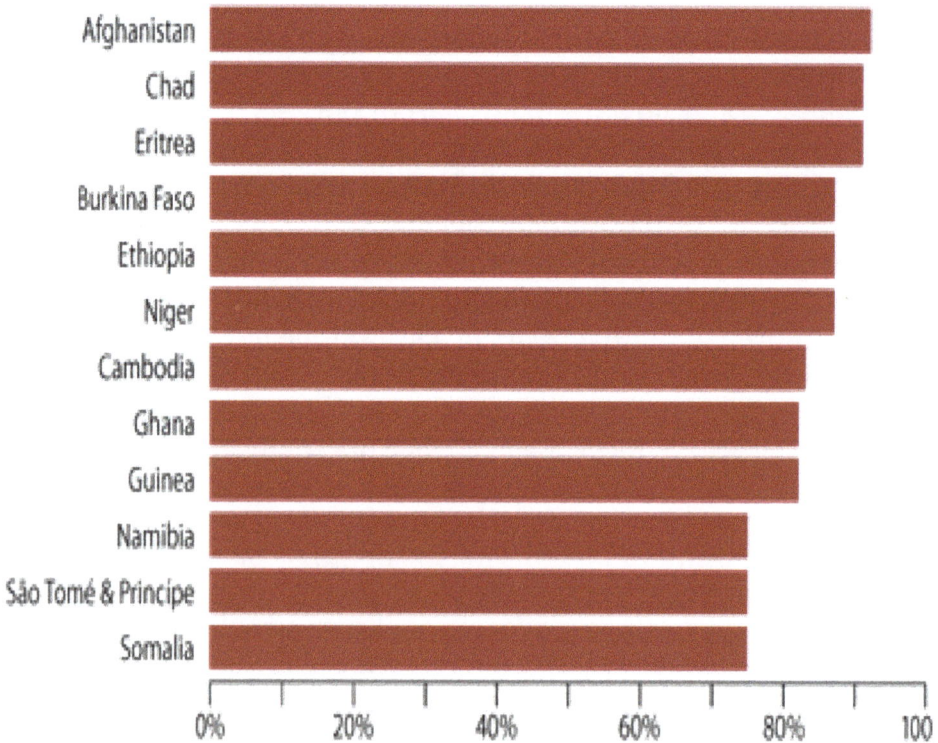

New Internationalist Magazine State of the World's Toilets, WaterAid based on data from WHO/UNICEF Joint Monitoring Programme.

Largest numbers of those without decent toilets by country[4]

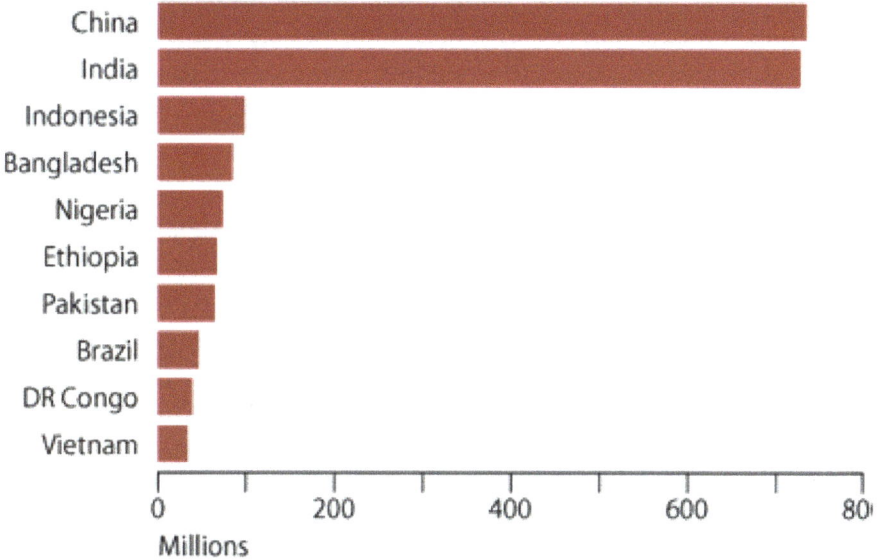

Country	
China	
India	
Indonesia	
Bangladesh	
Nigeria	
Ethiopia	
Pakistan	
Brazil	
DR Congo	
Vietnam	

0   200   400   600   80

Millions

New Internationalist Magazine State of the World's Toilets, WaterAid based on data from WHO/UNICEF Joint Monitoring Programme.

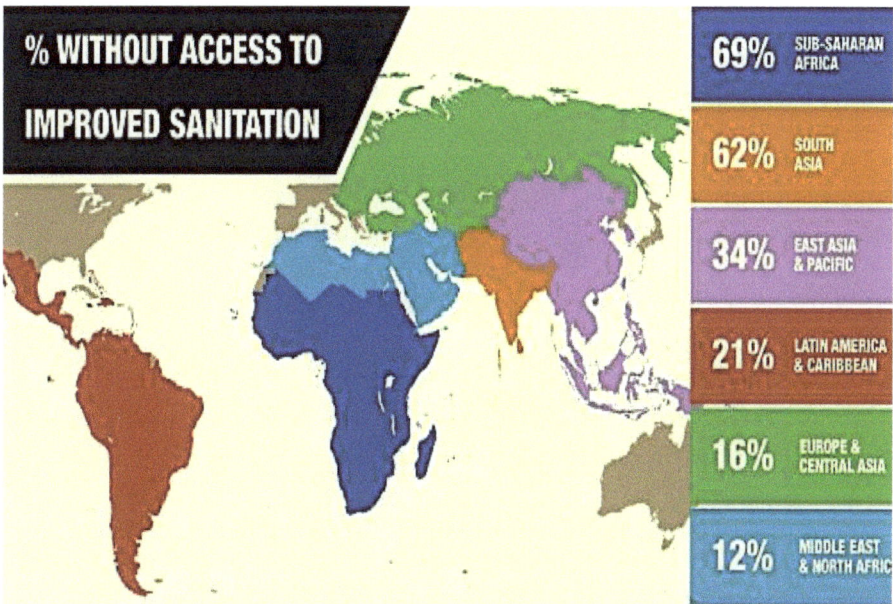

% WITHOUT ACCESS TO IMPROVED SANITATION

%	Region
69%	SUB-SAHARAN AFRICA
62%	SOUTH ASIA
34%	EAST ASIA & PACIFIC
21%	LATIN AMERICA & CARIBBEAN
16%	EUROPE & CENTRAL ASIA
12%	MIDDLE EAST & NORTH AFRICA

fastcompany.net Creative Commons License

Composting Toilet

A composting toilet is a dry toilet that uses managed aerobic decomposition to treat human waste. They are an alternative to flush toilets where there is a limited water supply or no waste treatment facility is available. The human excrement is normally mixed with sawdust, coconut coir, or peat moss to support aerobic processing, absorb liquids, and to reduce odor.

The decomposition process is typically faster than the anaerobic decomposition used in wet sewage systems such as septic tanks. Urine can contain ninety percent of the nitrogen, fifty percent of the phosphorus, and seventy percent of the potassium present in human excreta. In healthy individuals the urine is sterile and thus pathogen free. Undiluted urine may contain inorganic salts and organic compounds toxic to plants.

The requirement critical for aerobic microbial action is sufficient oxygen. Some units require manual methods for periodic aeration of the solid mass. Significant reductions in the volume of waste occur through the process with only ten percent of the inputs coming out as a humus-like material, which can be used as a soil amendment.

Pit Toilet

A pit toilet is a dry toilet system, which collects human excrement in a large container and can range from a simple slit trench to a more elaborate outhouse with a ventilation pipe. They are used in rural and wilderness areas as well as in much of the developing world. When the pit is improved with a small enclosed structure with a roof for shelter and a seat with a hole in it is commonly known as an outhouse.

The ventilated improved pit latrine, or VIP, is a pit toilet outhouse with a ventilation pipe and a screen at the top outlet. VIP latrines are an improvement over simple pit latrines by reducing odors, flies, and mosquitoes. nuisance and unpleasant odors. The ventilation pipe also removes the explosive danger of accumulated methane gas from the decomposition of the human waste in the pit.

Sewers

A sewage system may convey the wastewater by gravity, pumping, or vacuum to a sewage treatment plant. Pipelines range in size from six inches (150 mm) to tunnels of up to thirty feet (10 m) in diameter. Although sewer systems are intended to transport only sewage and not storm runoff all sewer systems have some degree of infiltration of groundwater, which can lead to sewer overflows.

The first sanitation system has been identified in prehistoric Ruins near Zabol, Iran. The ancient cities of Harappa and Mohenjo-Daro of the Indus Valley civilization developed networks of brick-lined sewers around 2600 BC and also had outdoor toilets that were flushed with water from reservoirs. Ancient Minoan civilization also had stone sewers that were flushed with water. Roman towns and garrisons in the United Kingdom between 46 BC and 400 AD had sewer networks sometimes constructed out of hollowed-out logs.

In the developed world sewers are usually pipelines from buildings to larger underground trunk mains, which transport the sewage to sewage treatment facilities. Vertical pipes, called manholes, connect the mains to the surface and are used for maintenance and to vent sewer gases. Sewers are generally gravity powered although pumping stations may be necessary. For decades sanitary sewer cracks or other damage could be repaired only by the expensive operation of digging up the damaged pipe and replacing it. In the mid-1950's technology advanced where a special cement mixture coated the inside of the pipe sealing all cracks and breaks.

Many cities built sewer systems to control outbreaks of disease such as typhoid and cholera. Initially these systems discharged sewage directly to surface waters such as rivers and lakes without treatment. As pollution of water bodies grew cities added sewage treatment plants to their systems to chlorinate and filter the water and sewage discharged. The institution of sewerage systems was a great public health advance.

Dung Beetle

Dung beetles are beetles that feed partly or exclusively on feces. All the species belong to the superfamily Scarabaeoidea, which alone comprises more than five thousand species. Many dung beetles known as 'rollers' roll dung into round balls, which are used as a food source or brooding chambers.

They can roll up to ten times their weight and some species can pull up to one thousand times their weight. Other dung beetles, known as tunnelers, bury the dung wherever they find it. A third group, the dwellers, neither roll nor burrow: they simply live in manure. Dung beetles are currently the only animals, other than humans, known to navigate and orient themselves using the Milky Way.

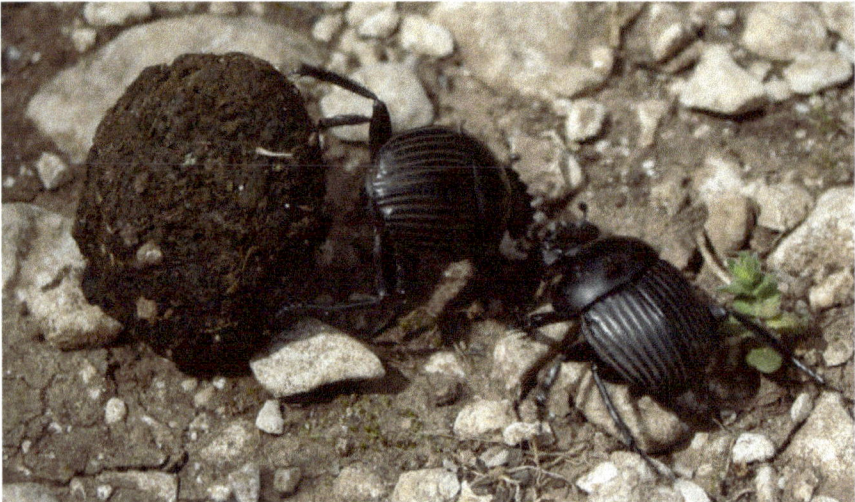

Scarabaeus iaticollis near a nuraghe near Monte Tiscali, Sardinia, Italy
Author Rafael Brix GNU Creative Commons

Dung beetles play an important role in agriculture. By burying and consuming dung they improve nutrient recycling and soil structure. They also protect livestock such as cattle by removing the dung, which if left in the open could provide habitat for pests. Many countries have introduced the creatures for the benefit of animal husbandry and as an adjunct for improving standards of hygiene.

Chamber Pot

A chamber pot (French: pot de chambre) is a pit like receptacle for receiving human waste. It was usually kept in the same chambers and under the sleeping bed, and since the sixteenth century often enclosed in a stool with a lid. Chamber pots were used in ancient Greece at least since the 6th century BC and remained in common use in many parts of the world until the mid-twentieth century. In rural areas lacking indoor plumbing they are still in use today. They have also been modified to serve as bedpans for the ill and disabled.

The affectionate term 'potty' is often used with children especially during toilet (potty) training. The term potty is also used to describe the child size chamber pot type toilets that are at the appropriate height for a child. Importantly, they also have a child size opening to sit on.

Regular adult toilets have an opening that is too large and frightening for a child who could accidentally fall in if not assisted. To remind you that their fear is not unjustified American adults suffer 40,000 toilet related injuries per year. Falling off a toilet directly contributed to the death of King George II of Great Britain. The height of the adult toilet does not allow their feet to touch the ground to assist in the squatting maneuver that assists defecation. A footstool to give their feet a place on which to rest can assist squatting, which eases the initiation of a bowel movement and can accelerate toilet training.

Close (Night) Stool

A close stool, also called a necessary or night stool, was in popular use for nearly five hundred years from the sixteenth century until the advent of indoor plumbing. It was an enclosed cabinet at chair height with an opening in the top often covered by a lid. It contained a pewter or earthenware chamber pot. In the nineteenth century it was referred to as a night commode, and in the twentieth century the commode euphemism was extended to the flush toilet.

Gong Farmer

Gong farmer was a term used in Tudor England for the worker who removed human excrement from outhouses, privies, cesspools, and cesspits. 'Gong' is derived from the Old English gang, which means 'to go', and since the eleventh century has been used to refer to a toilet facility, or privy, and its contents. They were only allowed to work at night and later became known as 'night soil men' or 'night man'. The human feces they collected were known as 'night soil' and were used as fertilizer. The emptying of cesspits today is usually accomplished with mechanical suction, by specialized tankers or trucks referred to by the euphemism Honey Truck or Honey Wagon.

Towns usually provided public latrines, known as houses of easement. Cesspits were often placed under cellar floors some of which had wooden chutes to convey the excrement. Cesspits allowed the liquid waste to drain leaving only the solids. Besides the offensive odor, cesspits were a continual problem as the accumulation of solid waste required the services of gong farmers to dig out and remove the excrement. Perhaps to avoid overfilling their cesspit it was not uncommon for the contents of chamber pots to be thrown into the streets from upstairs windows.

Despite being well paid, being a gong farmer was not considered an enviable occupation. They were only allowed to work between 9 PM and 5 AM and were permitted to live only in certain areas. Besides the occupational hazard of infectious diseases, concentrations of noxious and toxic gasses sometimes led to fatalities due to asphyxiation. Gong farmers often employed young boys to fill and lift buckets, known as a form of honey buckets, of excrement out of the pit because of the confined spaces. The excavated solid waste was removed in large barrels, which were loaded onto a horse-drawn cart called the honey cart or wagon. It was not an infrequent event to discover the corpse of an unwanted infant during the clearing of cesspits.

The job is still commonplace in India where it has estimated that up to 1.3 million Indians work with the collection of human waste. These workers are considered the lowest of the untouchable caste. They confine marriage to within its members leading to a waste-collecting caste passing the profession and caste burden on to the next generation. The film *Slumdog Millionaire* showed a brief glimpse of their existence.

Honey Bucket & Honey Wagon

A honey bucket is a bucket that is used as a toilet in locations that do not have more advanced facilities available. It often has a frame with a toilet seat lid and may be lined with a plastic bag for ease and convenience of disposal. A cover material such as sawdust may be used to reduce the odors from collected waste. Honey buckets are common in the far northern Arctic type climates especially where permafrost makes the installation of septic systems or outhouses impractical. They are seen throughout the world, especially in rural and undeveloped areas.

A honey wagon is a cart, wagon or truck for collecting and carrying excrement or manure. The term is often applied to the trucks that service septic tank systems as well as the bathroom on commercial aircraft. A recent news incident of a motor home bungled burglary was reminiscent of a honeywagon. The police were called to investigate what was presumed to be an attempt to siphon off and steal the gasoline from a parked vacation motor home. They found several empty gasoline transport containers, a length of rubber tubing, along with a pool of fecal material and vomited food. The nighttime would be fuel thieves opened the flap door, removed the cap, and put the siphon hose in an applied oral suction to start the flow of what they assume would be gasoline. The thieves opened the cap and valve to the septic system by mistake, got a mouthful of sewage, which they vomited up and fled the scene leaving their paraphernalia behind.

Night Soil

Night soil is the common name used for human fecal waste collected at night from cesspools and outhouses. It is often used as a fertilizer in developing countries where it contributes to the higher risk of acquiring parasites. This is not unexpected because the feces may well be contaminated and contain large quantities of parasite eggs, such as is commonly seen in the roundworm *Ascaris lumbricoides*. Rarely diseases have been transmitted into developed countries by the importation of vegetables with contaminated soil.

The use of night soil as fertilizer was common in Japan. The feces of rich people were sold at higher prices because their diet was better and it was thought that there would be more nutrients remaining in their waste. It brings a new level of understanding to the common phrases "filthy rich" and the "rich get richer".

Selling night soil as fertilizers became less common after World War II for sanitary reasons as well as the increased availability of chemical fertilizers. Modern Japan still has some areas with ongoing traditional night soil collection and disposal. The Japanese name for the 'outhouse within the house' style toilet, with the night soil collected, is Kumitori Benjo (汲み取り便所). China, Singapore, and Hong Kong also had extensive use of night soil collection, especially from urbanized areas where open honey buckets were carried through the streets. Hong Kong has a euphemism called 倒夜香, which literally means "pour night fragrant".

Septage

The partially treated waste in a septic tank that does not drain into the soil or is decomposed by the bacteria in the tank is called septage. This term should not be confused by a septuagenarian who in their 70's may occasionally feel like a septagenarian. It can be transported to local wastewater treatment centers or stored to be used as fertilizer.

The septage in a septic tank is usually considered in one of three categories. Scum which floats to the top generally harbor the greatest concentration of bacteria. The layer below is called the effluent and is a semi-treated liquid. The layer of solids at the bottom of the tank is called sludge. A septage pump truck removes the septage material from septic tanks, portable toilets, recreational vehicles such as motor homes, and boats. In commercial aviation and other industries, this type of vehicle may also be called a honey wagon, a reference to sewage collection of ages past.

Outhouse

Outhouses were popular before the advent of indoor plumbing. Because of the odor as well as flies and hygienic concerns, the deposit of human waste took place at a distance from the home. Many outhouses are simply holes in the ground, once the capacity is reached a new site is selected and the outhouse structure moved. To avoid the unpleasant odors, outhouses were usually kept a minimum of fifty feet away from a residence.

Keeping the waste site away from the source of drinking water is very important from a disease prevention and hygiene perspective. Many of the deaths attributed to military campaigns were actually caused by poor sanitation and waste management. The lack of hygiene and contaminated drinking water frequently led to more deaths and incapacitation of soldiers than those injured or killed in battles.

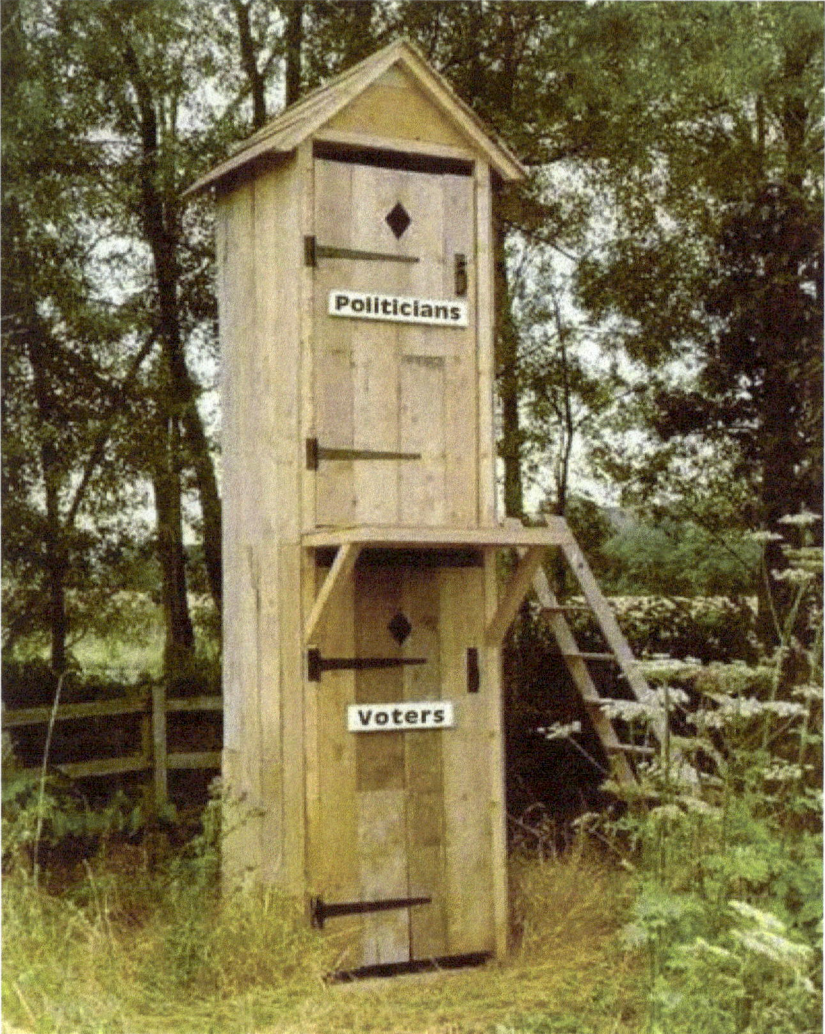

A two-story outhouse with a political satire message.

Toilet Gods

Deities associated with defecation and elimination have an ancient history preceding Babylonian times. They were worshipped in Roman times and still have a role in folk beliefs of indigenous peoples of Japan, China, New Zealand and other parts of the world. Such deities have been associated with bowel health, as well as general well-being and fertility because of the use of human waste as a fertilizer for agriculture.

Ancient Rome had three gods involved in the passage of human waste. The sewer goddess Cloacina (Latin sewer) had her origins in Etruscan beliefs and was the protector of the Cloaca Maxima, Rome's sewage system. Titus Tatius, who ruled early Rome with Romulus, built a shrine to her in his toilet and she was appealed to if sewers backed up. She was also the Goddess protector of sexual intercourse in marriage and her worship was later combined with that of Venus. Her image was placed on Roman coins.

Crepitus was described as the Roman god of flatulence but probably was a fiction created to denigrate Roman theology. He appears as a god in several works of French literature by Voltaire, Baudelaire, and Flaubert as well as material promoting Roman Catholicism as the true faith. Stercutius (Latin stercus 'excrement') was the god of dung who was particularly important to farmers when fertilizing their fields with manure. Worshipping the porcelain god, or ceramic throne, is a jocular reference to past toilet worship when heaving into the toilet bowl during vomiting.

Afterword

For those who are curious to know more about the physiology and science of the digestive process and intestinal gas several books in this series may be of interest. ***To 'Air' is Human, Everything You Ever Wanted to Know About Intestinal Gas*** covers everything you ever wanted to know about the burp, belch, bloat, fart and everything digestive, but were either too afraid or too embarrassed to ask. Intestinal gas has been produced and released by virtually every human who has ever lived, yet very few people have been provided with the knowledge that can offer comfort and relief. This volume is overflowing with practical information, fascinating facts, surprising trivia, and tasteful humorous insight about this universal phenomenon.

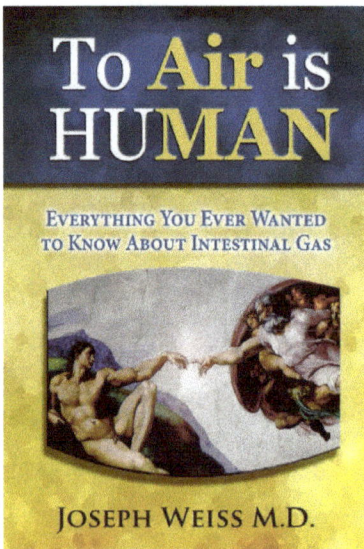

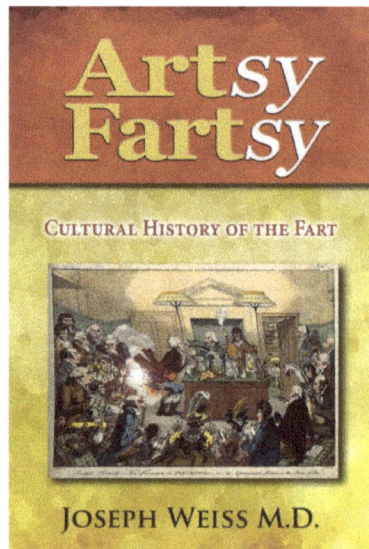

Artsy Fartsy, Cultural History of the Fart is a fascinating and factually correct review of the common fart through human culture and history. The cough, sneeze, hiccup, stomach rumble, burp, belch, and other bodily sounds simply cannot compete with the notoriety of the fart. Whether encountered live and in person or through the medium of literature, television, film, art, or music it may leave a powerful and lingering memory.

The Scoop on Poop! Flush with Knowledge is a uniquely informative tastefully entertaining, and well-illustrated volume that is full of it! The 'it' being a comprehensive and knowledgeable overview of all topics related to the remains of the digestive process. Whether you call it poop, feces, excrement, manure, dung, or the hundred plus other euphemisms, shit happens, and it happens a lot! Tens of billions of pounds and kilograms of it or deposited every day by while diversity of animal and microbial life. Humans alone contribute over three billion pounds a day, and only a small percentage of that is treated by a sewage system.

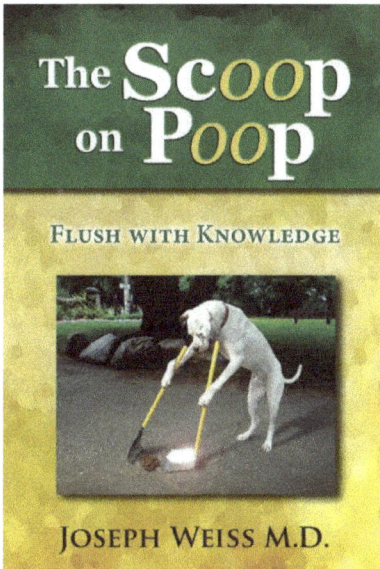

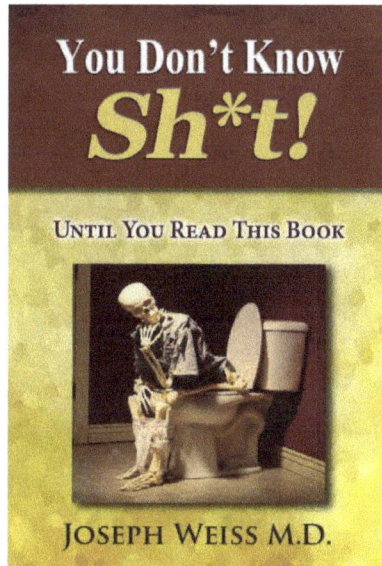

The identical content of The Scoop on Poop has been provocatively and cheekily retitled as ***You Don't Know Sh*t! Until You Read This Book***. This volume is an informative, entertaining and colorfully illustrated fountain of knowledge that is full of valuable information, including eccentricities and peculiarities, about the remains of the digestive process. Whether you disdain it, or appreciate it, it is part of the human (and animal) experience. The wealth of information and trivia can sustain a long social conversation, or cut it short abruptly!

AirVeda: Ancient & New Medical Wisdom, Digestion & Gas
covers the remarkable advances in the understanding of
digestive health and wellness. New information about the
critical role of genomics, epigenetics, the gut microbiome, and
the gut-brain-microbiome-diet axis are opening new avenues
to optimal whole body health and wellness. An appreciation of
the ancient wisdom of Ayurveda and other disciplines shows
that they had advanced insights into the nature of the human
body and the holistic approach.

*"Ayurveda is a 5,000 year old system of natural healing that
reminds us that health is the balanced and dynamic integration
between our environment, body, mind and spirit. In Dr. Joseph
Weiss' book, AirVeda, he provides an informative and
entertaining approach to sharing insights about our digestive
system and wellbeing by applying the ancient wisdom of
Ayurveda to everyday life."* **Deepak Chopra, MD**

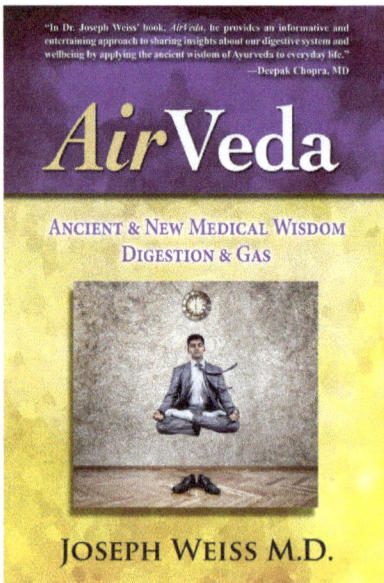

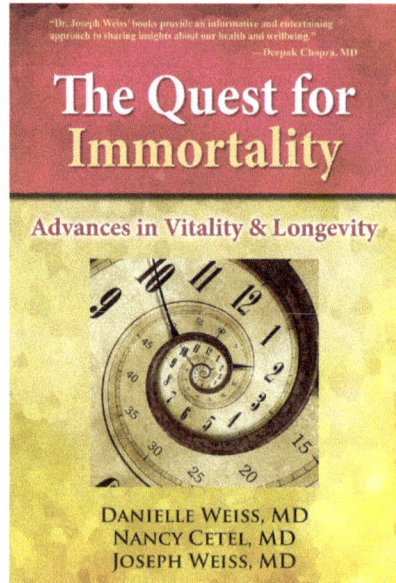

The Quest for Immortality, Advances in Vitality & Longevity
provides an informative and enlightening overview of the
remarkable advances in science and medicine that are
dramatically enhancing human health and lifespan. The volume

is written in clear, understandable, and engaging language with striking colorful illustrations. From groundbreaking nanotechnology to genomics and stem cells, the secrets of vitality and longevity are being uncovered along with more traditional advances and practical insights into disease prevention and health enhancement.

An even more comprehensive yet entertaining series are the extensive volumes of *Digestive Health & Disease, An Illustrated Encyclopedia of Everything You Ever Wanted to Know About Digestion & Nutrition*. These volumes are a uniquely informative, entertaining, and lavishly illustrated compendium of alimentary knowledge and eccentricities. It covers everything you ever wanted to know about digestion and nutrition in health and disease. Volumes One through Five are available on Amazon.com.

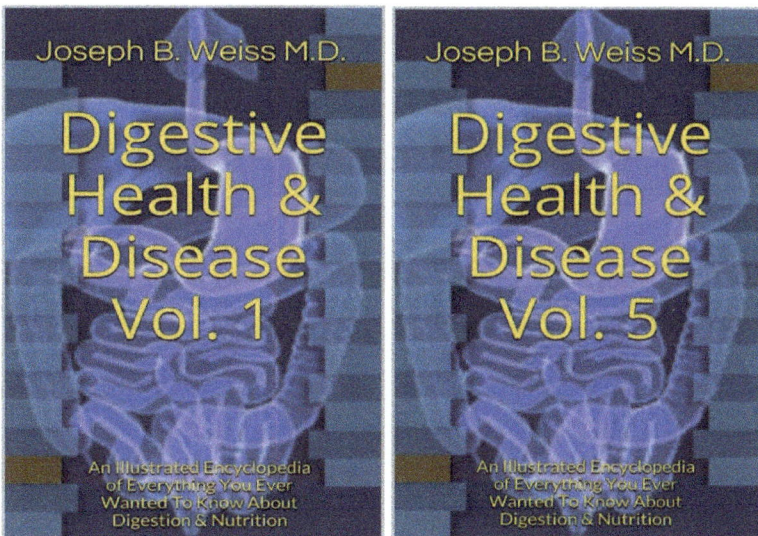

Organized as a reader friendly encyclopedia, the volumes cover over two thousand five hundred subject topics. Each volume may be utilized as an independent fully contained resource for the subjects it covers. The extensive size and scope of the series allows topics to be included that are rarely discussed in other books in the field and may be of great interest to the curious mind.

Written for the intelligent lay public, the medical and scientific terminology is translated into plain English. Practical and useful information and guidance are the primary goals, but entertaining and interesting information is included wherever possible. Designed for the visual learner as well, the clearly written text is supplemented by excellent photographs, illustrations, and charts. The reader will be informed, entertained, and the beneficiary of their newfound understanding of the universal process of digestion and metabolism that is the basis of all healthy living. The website www.smartaskbooks.com has a complete list of books and programs.